Little Miracles: A Comprehensive Guide to Pediatrics and Child Health

Welcome to "Little Miracles: A Comprehensive Guide to Pediatrics and Child Health." In this book, we embark on an extraordinary journey into the world of pediatrics, where we explore the fascinating realm of children's health and well-being. From the moment a child takes their first breath to the complexities of adolescence, pediatric care plays a vital role in nurturing and safeguarding these little miracles.

As parents, caregivers, and healthcare professionals, understanding the unique needs of children is paramount to providing them with the best possible care. The goal of this book is to empower you with knowledge and insights that will enable you to navigate the joys and challenges of raising healthy and happy children.

Throughout these pages, we will delve into various aspects of pediatric healthcare, starting with the basics of general pediatrics, including child growth and development, preventive care, and immunizations. We will explore common childhood illnesses and how to manage them, as well as allergies, asthma, and other prevalent conditions affecting children.

Emergencies can strike when least expected, so we will equip you with essential knowledge on recognizing and responding to pediatric emergencies, including first aid techniques and basic life support.

Additionally, we will delve into perinatology and neonatology, shedding light on the early stages of life, prenatal care, and the specialized care offered in neonatal intensive care units (NICUs). Understanding newborn care, breastfeeding, and infant nutrition is essential to give our little ones the best start in life.

As we journey through childhood, we will address nutrition, childhood development, and behavior, offering guidance on building healthy eating habits, managing picky eaters, and addressing behavioral challenges. We will also touch on developmental milestones, autism spectrum disorder, and developmental delays.

Specialty care is an integral part of pediatric medicine, so we will explore various pediatric subspecialties, including cardiology, pulmonology, neurology, gastroenterology, and oncology.

Chronic conditions in children can be challenging for families, and we will discuss diabetes, endocrine disorders, and how to support families facing long-term care needs.

Child mental health and emotional well-being are critical aspects of pediatric care, and we will provide insights into recognizing and addressing childhood anxiety, depression, trauma, and building resilience.

Safety is of utmost importance, so we will delve into childproofing, accident prevention, and child safety measures to ensure a secure environment for children.

As children transition into adolescence, we will explore the unique health needs of teenagers, including puberty, mental health, and substance abuse.

The book will also cover child mental health and emotional well-being, addressing childhood anxiety, depression, and trauma, while also emphasizing building resilience in children.

Child health is a global endeavor, and we will look at child health issues worldwide, including healthcare advancements and challenges, with a focus on ensuring a healthy future for children everywhere.

Our little miracles are our future, and caring for them is a privilege and responsibility. This book aims to empower parents, caregivers, and healthcare professionals with knowledge and tools to provide the best care for the little miracles in their lives. As we journey through the world of pediatrics together, may this guide be a beacon of knowledge and support, fostering a healthier and happier world for our little miracles.

I. Introduction to Pediatrics

- Welcome to the World of Pediatrics
- The Role of Pediatricians in Child Health

II. General Pediatrics

- Child Growth and Development
- Pediatric Preventive Care and Well-Child Visits
- Immunizations and Vaccine Schedules
- Common Childhood Illnesses and Infections
- Allergies and Asthma in Children

III. Pediatric Emergencies

- Recognizing and Responding to Pediatric Emergencies
- First Aid for Common Childhood Injuries
- Pediatric CPR and Basic Life Support
- Managing Pediatric Emergencies at Home and in the Community

IV. Perinatology and Neonatology

- Prenatal Care and Antenatal Screening

- High-Risk Pregnancy and Maternal Health
- Neonatal Care and the Neonatal Intensive Care Unit (NICU)
- Common Neonatal Conditions and Prematurity

V. Newborn Care and Infant Health

- The First Days of Life: Newborn Care and Adaptation
- Breastfeeding and Infant Nutrition
- Infant Sleep and Caring for Sleep-Deprived Parents
- Infant Developmental Milestones

VI. Childhood Nutrition and Feeding

- Nutritional Needs of Infants, Toddlers, and Children
- Healthy Eating Habits for Children
- Managing Picky Eaters and Food Allergies

VII. Childhood Development and Behavior

- Cognitive, Social, and Emotional Development
- Behavioral Challenges and Discipline Strategies
- Autism Spectrum Disorder and Developmental Delays

VIII. Pediatric Specialty Care

- Pediatric Cardiology: Heart Health in Children
- Pediatric Pulmonology: Respiratory Health in Children
- Pediatric Neurology: Brain and Nervous System Health
- Pediatric Gastroenterology: Digestive Health in Children
- Pediatric Oncology: Childhood Cancer Care

IX. Chronic Conditions and Long-Term Care

- Empowering Parents and Caregivers in Child Health
- Encouragement for Further Exploration and Advocacy for Child Health

Welcome to the World of Pediatrics

Thank you! Pediatrics is a fascinating field that deals with the medical care of infants, children, and adolescents. Pediatricians play a crucial role in ensuring the health and well-being of young patients, monitoring their growth and development, diagnosing and treating illnesses, and providing preventive care.

Working in pediatrics requires not only medical knowledge and expertise but also a compassionate and patient-centered approach. Children can present unique challenges in healthcare, and it's essential for pediatricians to have excellent communication skills to interact with both their young patients and their parents or guardians.

Pediatric medicine encompasses a wide range of specialties, including neonatology for newborns, pediatric cardiology for heart-related conditions, pediatric oncology for childhood cancers, and many others. As medical knowledge advances, so does the ability to improve the quality of care provided to children.

It's a rewarding and fulfilling field, knowing that you are making a difference in the lives of young patients and helping them to grow up healthy and happy.

The Role of Pediatricians in Child Health

Pediatricians play a critical role in child health, as they are specialized doctors trained to care for infants, children, and adolescents. Their role extends from providing routine check-ups and vaccinations to diagnosing and treating various medical conditions that affect children. Here are some key aspects of their role in child health:

1. Preventive Care: Pediatricians focus on preventive care, emphasizing the importance of regular check-ups and vaccinations to protect children from preventable diseases. They monitor a child's growth and development and offer guidance on nutrition, exercise, and safety to promote overall well-being.

2. Diagnosis and Treatment: When a child is sick or experiencing health issues, pediatricians are trained to diagnose and treat a wide range of medical conditions. They can address common childhood illnesses such as ear infections, respiratory infections, and allergies, as well as more complex conditions like asthma, diabetes, and childhood cancers.

3. Developmental Screening: Pediatricians conduct developmental screenings to identify any delays or issues in a child's physical, cognitive, or behavioral development. Early detection and intervention are crucial in addressing developmental delays and providing appropriate support.

4. Parental Guidance: Pediatricians provide guidance and

support to parents and caregivers in various aspects of child-rearing, including feeding, sleep, behavior management, and safety. They serve as a reliable resource for parents to address their concerns and questions about their child's health.

5. Managing Chronic Conditions: For children with chronic medical conditions or special healthcare needs, pediatricians play a vital role in managing their ongoing care, coordinating with other specialists, and ensuring a comprehensive and holistic approach to treatment.

6. Advocacy: Pediatricians advocate for the health and well-being of children at individual, community, and policy levels. They may participate in public health campaigns, raise awareness about child health issues, and work to implement policies that benefit children's health.

7. Emotional Support: Pediatricians are sensitive to the emotional needs of both children and parents during times of illness or medical treatment. They strive to create a supportive and caring environment to help children and families cope with medical challenges.

8. Research and Education: Many pediatricians are involved in research to advance medical knowledge in the field of child health. They also play a crucial role in educating medical students, residents, and other healthcare professionals about pediatric care and child development.

Overall, pediatricians are dedicated to the health and well-being of children and are instrumental in ensuring that the youngest members of society receive the best possible medical care and support.

Child Growth and Development

Child growth and development refer to the physical, cognitive, emotional, and social changes that occur as a child progresses from infancy to adolescence. It is a complex and continuous process influenced by genetic, environmental, and socio-cultural factors. Understanding child growth and development is crucial for parents, caregivers, educators, and healthcare professionals to provide appropriate support and promote optimal development. Here are the key stages of child growth and development:

1. Infancy (0-2 years): Infancy is a period of rapid growth and development. During this stage, infants go through significant physical changes, such as gaining weight, growing in length, and developing motor skills like crawling, sitting, and walking. They also experience cognitive development, becoming more aware of their surroundings, and forming attachments to caregivers. Language development begins as infants coo, babble, and eventually say their first words.

2. Early Childhood (2-6 years): This stage is characterized by continued physical growth and the refinement of motor skills. Children's language skills expand, and they become more curious and imaginative. They also develop social skills and learn to interact and play with others. Early childhood is a critical period for the development of basic cognitive abilities, such as problem-solving, memory, and concentration.

3. Middle Childhood (6-12 years): Middle childhood is a time of steady physical growth and the development of more refined motor skills. Children's cognitive abilities

further mature, allowing for more complex thinking and reasoning. Socially, they develop friendships and start to understand social norms and rules. Emotional regulation and self-awareness also improve during this stage.

4. Adolescence (12-18 years): Adolescence is a period of significant physical and hormonal changes, marking the transition from childhood to adulthood. Puberty begins, leading to the development of secondary sexual characteristics and increased growth spurts. Cognitive development during adolescence involves more sophisticated thinking, abstract reasoning, and long-term planning. Socially, adolescents seek greater independence from their families and form stronger peer relationships. They also develop their identities and moral values.

It's essential to recognize that each child develops at their own pace, and there can be variations in individual development. Some children may reach certain milestones earlier or later than others. Early intervention and support can be beneficial if there are concerns about a child's growth and development.

Parents and caregivers can support healthy child growth and development by providing a nurturing and stimulating environment, engaging in age-appropriate activities, ensuring proper nutrition and healthcare, and being responsive to their emotional needs. Regular check-ups with pediatricians and educators can also help monitor developmental progress and address any concerns promptly.

Pediatric Preventive Care and Well-Child Visits

Pediatric preventive care and well-child visits are essential components of promoting the health and well-being of children. Preventive care focuses on early detection, prevention, and intervention to ensure that children stay healthy and reach their full potential. Well-child visits are regular check-ups with a pediatrician or healthcare provider that are scheduled at specific intervals throughout a child's early years. Here's an overview of pediatric preventive care and well-child visits:

1. Purpose of Well-Child Visits: Well-child visits are scheduled at various ages and are designed to monitor a child's growth and development, provide vaccinations, conduct screenings, and address any health concerns or questions parents may have. These visits also give healthcare providers the opportunity to build a relationship with the child and their family, which can lead to better communication and understanding of the child's healthcare needs.

2. Components of Well-Child Visits: During well-child visits, pediatricians typically perform a comprehensive physical examination, including measurements of height, weight, and head circumference to track growth patterns. Developmental milestones are assessed to ensure the child is meeting age-appropriate developmental targets. Vaccinations are administered based on the recommended immunization schedule. Hearing and vision screenings are often conducted.

Nutrition and safety issues may also be discussed.

3. Early Detection and Prevention: Well-child visits are an essential part of early detection and prevention of health problems. Regular screenings and assessments can identify any developmental delays, behavioral concerns, or medical conditions early on, allowing for timely intervention and appropriate treatment.

4. Vaccinations: Well-child visits are the primary occasions for administering vaccinations according to the recommended immunization schedule. Vaccinations protect children from serious and potentially life-threatening diseases and contribute to the overall health of the community through herd immunity.

5. Parental Guidance and Education: Well-child visits provide an opportunity for pediatricians to offer guidance and education to parents and caregivers on various aspects of child health, nutrition, safety, behavior, and development. Parental involvement is crucial in maintaining a child's health and well-being.

6. Building a Medical Home: Regular well-child visits establish a medical home for the child—a consistent and continuous source of healthcare that promotes personalized, family-centered care. This medical home helps coordinate care and ensures comprehensive healthcare services for the child.

7. Schedule of Well-Child Visits: The schedule of well-child visits may vary slightly depending on the healthcare provider and the child's specific needs. Generally, well-child visits are recommended at birth, 1-2 weeks, 1, 2, 4, 6, 9, 12, 15, 18, and 24 months, and then annually during childhood and adolescence.

By attending well-child visits and following recommended preventive care guidelines, parents and caregivers can play an active role in maintaining the health and well-being of their children, while pediatricians can provide early intervention and support to ensure optimal child development.

Immunizations and Vaccine Schedules

Immunizations, also known as vaccinations or vaccines, are crucial in protecting individuals from infectious diseases by stimulating the immune system to produce antibodies against specific pathogens. Vaccines have been instrumental in preventing the spread of various serious and potentially life-threatening diseases, saving millions of lives worldwide. Here's an overview of immunizations and vaccine schedules:

1. Importance of Immunizations: Immunizations are essential because they help prevent the spread of infectious diseases, protect vulnerable populations (such as infants, elderly individuals, and individuals with weakened immune systems), and contribute to herd immunity. Herd immunity occurs when a significant portion of the population is vaccinated, making it harder for the disease to spread, thereby protecting those who cannot be vaccinated.

2. Vaccine Schedule: The vaccine schedule is a recommended timeline of when vaccines should be administered to children and adults. The schedule is designed to provide protection against diseases at the most vulnerable age groups and to ensure the most effective immune response.

3. Childhood Immunization Schedule: In many countries, including the United States, childhood immunization schedules are developed and maintained by national health authorities. The schedule typically starts at birth and continues through adolescence. It includes vaccines for diseases such as measles, mumps, rubella,

diphtheria, tetanus, pertussis (whooping cough), polio, hepatitis B, varicella (chickenpox), and many others.

4. Adult Immunization Schedule: Immunizations are not just for children; adults also need vaccinations to protect themselves and those around them. The adult immunization schedule includes vaccines for diseases like influenza (flu), pneumococcal disease, shingles, and tetanus, among others.

5. Recommended Catch-up Vaccination: If a child or adult misses one or more vaccinations according to the recommended schedule, a catch-up vaccination plan may be recommended by a healthcare provider. This helps ensure that individuals are adequately protected against preventable diseases.

6. Vaccine Safety: Vaccines undergo rigorous testing and evaluation for safety and efficacy before they are approved for use. The benefits of vaccination far outweigh the risks, and serious side effects are rare. Common side effects may include mild fever or soreness at the injection site.

7. Travel Vaccinations: When traveling to certain regions, additional vaccinations may be recommended to protect against specific diseases that are prevalent in those areas.

It is essential to follow the recommended vaccine schedule and to consult with healthcare providers to ensure that individuals receive all necessary vaccinations. Maintaining high vaccination rates within a population is critical in preventing outbreaks of vaccine-preventable diseases and protecting public health.

Common Childhood Illnesses and Infections

Children are susceptible to various illnesses and infections due to their developing immune systems and exposure to new environments. Many of these illnesses are common in childhood and are generally mild and self-limiting. Some of the most common childhood illnesses and infections include:

1. Common Cold: The common cold is a viral infection that causes symptoms such as a runny or stuffy nose, sneezing, coughing, and mild fever. It is highly contagious and spreads through respiratory droplets.
2. Influenza (Flu): The flu is a viral respiratory infection that can cause fever, chills, body aches, cough, sore throat, and fatigue. It is more severe than the common cold and can lead to complications in young children.
3. Gastroenteritis: Gastroenteritis, often called the stomach flu, is an infection of the stomach and intestines, usually caused by viruses or bacteria. It leads to symptoms such as vomiting, diarrhea, abdominal cramps, and dehydration.
4. Ear Infections: Ear infections are common in children, especially those between 6 months and 2 years old. They occur when bacteria or viruses cause inflammation in the middle ear, leading to ear pain and sometimes fever.
5. Streptococcal Pharyngitis (Strep Throat): Strep throat is a bacterial infection caused by Group A Streptococcus bacteria. It results in a sore throat, difficulty swallowing, fever, and sometimes a rash.

6. Hand, Foot, and Mouth Disease (HFMD): HFMD is a viral infection common in young children. It causes sores in the mouth and a rash on the hands and feet, along with fever and general discomfort.

7. Chickenpox: Chickenpox is a highly contagious viral infection caused by the varicella-zoster virus. It results in a red, itchy rash and fever. Most children recover without complications, but it can be more severe in adolescents and adults.

8. Measles: Measles is a highly contagious viral infection characterized by a high fever, cough, runny nose, and a distinctive red rash. It can lead to severe complications, especially in unvaccinated individuals.

9. Croup: Croup is a viral infection that causes inflammation of the upper airways, leading to a barking cough, hoarseness, and difficulty breathing.

10. Roseola: Roseola, or sixth disease, is a viral infection that causes high fever followed by a rash. The fever often subsides before the rash appears.

It's essential for parents and caregivers to be aware of the signs and symptoms of these common childhood illnesses and infections. Most of these conditions can be managed at home with rest, fluids, and over-the-counter medications for symptom relief. However, if a child's symptoms are severe, persistent, or accompanied by concerning signs, it's important to seek medical attention promptly. Vaccination is a key preventive measure against many of these illnesses and can help protect children from serious complications.

Allergies and Asthma in Children

Allergies and asthma are common chronic conditions that can affect children, often beginning in early childhood or during the school-age years. Both allergies and asthma are related to the immune system's response to specific triggers, but they have distinct characteristics and symptoms. Here's an overview of allergies and asthma in children:

Allergies in Children:

1. Allergic Reactions: Allergies occur when a child's immune system overreacts to substances that are typically harmless, such as pollen, pet dander, mold spores, dust mites, certain foods, or insect stings. When exposed to these triggers, the immune system releases chemicals, such as histamines, leading to allergic reactions.

2. Common Allergy Symptoms: Allergy symptoms can vary depending on the allergen and the child's sensitivity. Common symptoms include sneezing, runny or stuffy nose, itchy and watery eyes, skin rashes (like hives), itching, and sometimes asthma-like symptoms, such as coughing and wheezing.

3. Allergic Asthma: Some children with allergies may develop allergic asthma, where exposure to allergens triggers inflammation and constriction of the airways, leading to asthma symptoms like coughing, wheezing, shortness of breath, and chest tightness.

Asthma in Children:

1. Asthma is a chronic respiratory condition characterized by inflammation and narrowing of the airways, making it difficult for a child to breathe. Asthma symptoms can be triggered by various factors, including allergens, respiratory infections, exercise, cold air, and irritants like tobacco smoke.
2. Common Asthma Symptoms: Asthma symptoms in children include coughing (especially at night or with exercise), wheezing (a high-pitched whistling sound when breathing out), shortness of breath, and chest tightness.
3. Asthma Triggers: In addition to allergens, asthma triggers can include respiratory infections, tobacco smoke, air pollution, cold air, strong odors or fumes, and emotional stress.

Management and Treatment:

1. Allergy Management: Identifying and avoiding allergens is an essential part of managing allergies. Antihistamines and nasal corticosteroid sprays may be prescribed to relieve allergy symptoms. In severe cases, allergen immunotherapy (allergy shots) may be recommended to desensitize the child's immune system to specific allergens.
2. Asthma Management: Asthma management involves long-term control and quick-relief medications. Long-term control medications, such as inhaled corticosteroids, help reduce airway inflammation, while quick-relief medications (bronchodilators) provide rapid relief during asthma attacks. An asthma action plan helps parents and caregivers monitor and respond to a child's asthma symptoms effectively.

It is essential for parents and caregivers of children with allergies or asthma to work closely with healthcare providers to develop a comprehensive management plan tailored to the child's specific needs. Regular follow-up visits with a pediatrician or pediatric allergist/immunologist can help monitor symptoms, adjust treatment plans, and ensure optimal asthma and allergy control for the child's overall health and well-being.

Recognizing and Responding to Pediatric Emergencies

Recognizing and responding to pediatric emergencies promptly and appropriately is crucial in ensuring the best possible outcomes for children in critical situations. Pediatric emergencies can arise from various causes, including accidents, sudden illnesses, allergic reactions, respiratory distress, and more. Here are some important steps to recognize and respond to pediatric emergencies:

1. Stay Calm: In any emergency situation involving a child, it is vital for adults to remain calm. Panicking can hinder clear thinking and quick decision-making, so take a deep breath and try to stay composed.

2. Assess the Situation: Quickly assess the child's condition and the nature of the emergency. Check for responsiveness, breathing, and circulation. If the child is unresponsive and not breathing or only gasping, immediate cardiopulmonary resuscitation (CPR) is necessary.

3. Call for Help: If the situation requires immediate medical attention, call emergency services or the local emergency number (e.g., 911 in the United States) to request professional medical assistance.

4. Start CPR (if needed): If the child is unresponsive and not breathing or only gasping, begin CPR immediately. If you are trained in CPR, initiate chest compressions and rescue breaths. Continue CPR until emergency medical help arrives.

5. Control Bleeding: In cases of significant bleeding, apply direct pressure to the wound with a clean cloth or sterile dressing to control bleeding. Elevate the injured limb if possible.

6. Support Breathing: If a child is experiencing breathing difficulties or choking, encourage them to cough forcefully if conscious. For choking infants or conscious children who cannot cough, perform the Heimlich maneuver appropriately.

7. Administer Epinephrine (if prescribed): For children with severe allergic reactions (anaphylaxis) and prescribed epinephrine auto-injectors, promptly administer the epinephrine as instructed.

8. Avoid Delay: In a pediatric emergency, time is of the essence. Avoid unnecessary delays in seeking medical help and follow appropriate protocols for first aid and emergency response.

9. Communicate Clearly: Provide clear and concise information to emergency responders about the child's condition, any known allergies or medical conditions, and any actions taken.

10. Stay With the Child: If you are not alone, assign someone to stay with the child while others call for help or retrieve necessary supplies.

It is essential to be prepared for pediatric emergencies by learning basic first aid and CPR techniques. Additionally, having a basic understanding of common pediatric emergencies and their warning signs can help parents, caregivers, and teachers recognize when a child needs immediate medical attention. Regular safety measures and preventive strategies can also reduce the risk of accidents and emergencies involving children. Always seek immediate professional medical attention for any concerning or life-threatening situation involving a child.

First Aid for Common Childhood Injuries

First aid for common childhood injuries is essential knowledge for parents, caregivers, teachers, and anyone responsible for the well-being of children. Here are some first aid steps for common childhood injuries:

1. Cuts and Scrapes:
   - Clean the wound gently with mild soap and water.
   - Apply gentle pressure with a clean cloth to stop bleeding.
   - Cover the wound with a sterile bandage or dressing to protect it from infection.

2. Burns:
   - For minor burns, run cool (not cold) water over the affected area for at least 10 minutes to reduce heat and pain.
   - Cover the burn with a sterile, non-stick dressing.
   - Seek medical attention for more severe burns, burns on the face, hands, feet, or genitals, or burns caused by chemicals or electricity.

3. Bruises:
   - Apply a cold compress or ice pack wrapped in a cloth to the bruised area to reduce swelling and pain.
   - If there is significant pain or swelling, or if the child is unable to move the injured area, seek

medical attention.

4. Sprains and Strains:
   - RICE method: Rest the injured area, apply Ice to reduce swelling, compress the area with an elastic bandage, and elevate the injured limb to reduce swelling further.
   - Avoid putting weight on the injured limb and seek medical attention if there is severe pain, swelling, or inability to move the limb.

5. Nosebleeds:
   - Have the child sit upright and lean forward slightly.
   - Pinch the soft part of the nose (not the bony part) with fingers for about 10 minutes while breathing through the mouth.
   - If the bleeding persists or is severe, seek medical attention.

6. Insect Bites and Stings:
   - Remove the stinger if present by scraping it off with a flat object (e.g., credit card).
   - Clean the affected area with soap and water.
   - Apply a cold compress to reduce swelling and itching.
   - If the child shows signs of an allergic reaction (difficulty breathing, hives, swelling of the face or throat), seek emergency medical help.

7. Head Injuries:
   - For minor bumps or falls without loss of consciousness, apply a cold compress to the affected area to reduce swelling.
   - If there is a loss of consciousness, vomiting, confusion, or any other concerning symptoms, seek immediate medical attention.

8. Choking:
   - For conscious choking, perform the Heimlich maneuver appropriately based on the child's

      age and size.

- If the child becomes unconscious, start CPR and continue until emergency help arrives.

Remember that these are general first aid guidelines for common childhood injuries. If a child's injury is severe, if there are signs of a more serious condition, or if you are unsure how to handle the situation, seek professional medical help promptly. Taking a certified first aid course can provide valuable skills and knowledge in handling a wide range of childhood emergencies safely and effectively.

Pediatric CPR and Basic Life Support

Pediatric CPR (Cardiopulmonary Resuscitation) and Basic Life Support (BLS) are essential life-saving techniques used to revive a child who is experiencing cardiac arrest or is unresponsive and not breathing. Prompt and effective CPR can make a significant difference in improving the chances of survival for a child in a life-threatening emergency. Here are the basic steps for pediatric CPR and BLS:

1. Check for Responsiveness: First, assess the child's responsiveness by tapping the child and shouting loudly to see if they respond.
2. Call for Help: If the child is unresponsive and not breathing or only gasping, call emergency services or the local emergency number (e.g., 911 in the United States) immediately to request professional medical assistance.
3. Start Chest Compressions:
   - Place the child on their back on a firm, flat surface.
   - For infants (up to age 1):
     - Locate the correct hand position: Use two fingers (index and middle fingers) to compress the center of the chest, just below the nipple line.
     - Compress the chest about 1.5 inches (approximately 1/3 of the depth of the chest) at a rate of about 100-120

compressions per minute.
- For children (age 1 to puberty):
  - Use the heel of one or both hands to compress the center of the chest, just below the nipple line.
  - Compress the chest about 2 inches at a rate of about 100-120 compressions per minute.
- Allow the chest to fully recoil between compressions without lifting your hands off the chest.

4. Give Rescue Breaths (if trained and comfortable to do so):
- After 30 compressions, open the child's airway by tilting the head backward and lifting the chin.
- Pinch the child's nose closed and give two gentle breaths (1 second each) into the child's mouth, making sure to see the chest rise with each breath.
- Continue with cycles of 30 compressions and 2 breaths until help arrives, the child starts breathing on their own, or you are too exhausted to continue.

Remember these important points while performing pediatric CPR and BLS:

- Push hard and fast: Compress the chest firmly and at an adequate rate.
- Minimize interruptions: Avoid extended pauses during CPR.
- Avoid excessive ventilation: Give just enough breaths to see the chest rise.

It is essential to learn and practice pediatric CPR and BLS techniques through certified training courses. The American

Heart Association (AHA) and the American Red Cross offer pediatric CPR and BLS courses that provide hands-on training and guidance on performing CPR safely and effectively on infants and children. Having the skills and confidence to perform pediatric CPR can be lifesaving in critical situations involving children.

Managing Pediatric Emergencies at Home and in the Community

Managing pediatric emergencies at home and in the community involves being prepared, staying calm, and taking prompt and appropriate actions to ensure the safety and well-being of the child. Here are some essential steps for managing pediatric emergencies:

1. Prevention:
   - The best way to manage emergencies is to prevent them whenever possible. Take safety measures at home and in the community, such as using safety gates, securing furniture, wearing helmets, using car seats and seat belts correctly, and practicing water safety.
2. First Aid Training:
   - Parents, caregivers, and older children should consider taking certified first aid and CPR courses. Proper training equips individuals with essential life-saving skills to handle emergencies confidently and effectively.
3. Stay Calm and Assess the Situation:
   - In an emergency, staying calm is crucial. Assess the child's condition and surroundings to determine the appropriate response.
4. Call for Help:
   - If the situation requires immediate medical attention, call emergency services or the local emergency number (e.g., 911 in the

United States) to request professional medical assistance.

5. Provide First Aid:
   - Administer first aid as necessary based on the specific emergency. This may include performing CPR, controlling bleeding, managing burns, providing rescue breaths, and immobilizing suspected fractures.
6. Involve Bystanders:
   - If there are bystanders, delegate specific tasks to them, such as calling for help, gathering first aid supplies, or comforting the child.
7. Communicate Clearly:
   - Provide clear and concise information to emergency responders about the child's condition, any known allergies or medical conditions, and any actions taken.
8. Follow Emergency Action Plans:
   - If the child has known medical conditions or allergies, be familiar with their emergency action plan and follow it accordingly.
9. Stay with the Child:
   - Stay with the child and provide comfort and reassurance until professional medical help arrives.
10. Activate Emergency Medical Alert:
    - If the child has a medical alert bracelet or necklace, make sure to activate it to provide crucial medical information to first responders.
11. Prevent Choking Hazards:
    - Keep small objects, toys, and food items that can pose a choking hazard out of reach of young children.

Remember that immediate medical attention may be required for certain emergencies, and first aid is only the initial response until professional medical help arrives. It's essential to call for help early and avoid delays in seeking professional medical attention for pediatric emergencies. Being prepared and having the knowledge and skills to respond to emergencies can make a significant difference in the outcome of a pediatric emergency at home or in the community.

Prenatal Care and Antenatal Screening

Prenatal care and antenatal screening are essential components of healthcare for pregnant women. Prenatal care focuses on monitoring the health of the mother and the developing fetus during pregnancy to ensure a healthy pregnancy and delivery. Antenatal screening involves a series of tests and assessments to identify and manage potential health risks for both the mother and the baby. Here's an overview of prenatal care and antenatal screening:

Prenatal Care:

1. Early Initiation: Prenatal care typically begins as soon as a woman confirms her pregnancy, preferably within the first trimester (first 12 weeks of pregnancy). Early initiation allows for timely interventions and proper management of any potential health issues.
2. Regular Check-ups: Throughout pregnancy, expectant mothers should have regular check-ups with a healthcare provider. The frequency of visits may vary depending on the woman's health, the complexity of the pregnancy, and any pre-existing medical conditions.
3. Physical Examinations: During prenatal visits, healthcare providers conduct physical examinations to monitor the mother's overall health, blood pressure, weight gain, and fetal growth.
4. Blood and Urine Tests: Blood and urine tests are commonly performed during prenatal care to check for conditions such as anemia, gestational diabetes, and urinary tract infections.
5. Fetal Monitoring: Fetal heartbeat and growth are

regularly monitored using techniques like ultrasound scans, Doppler ultrasound, or electronic fetal monitoring.

6. Nutrition and Lifestyle Guidance: Prenatal care includes guidance on proper nutrition, exercise, and lifestyle choices, such as avoiding alcohol, tobacco, and certain medications that may pose risks during pregnancy.

7. Education and Counseling: Expectant mothers receive information on pregnancy, childbirth, breastfeeding, and postpartum care. They are also counseled on birth control options and family planning after delivery.

Antenatal Screening:

1. Genetic Screening: Genetic screening tests, such as carrier screening and non-invasive prenatal testing (NIPT), can assess the risk of the baby having certain genetic conditions, such as Down syndrome, trisomy 18, and neural tube defects.

2. Blood Tests: Blood tests may be performed to screen for conditions like gestational diabetes, anemia, and certain infections that can affect pregnancy.

3. Ultrasound Scans: Ultrasound scans are used to assess fetal development, check for abnormalities, and estimate gestational age.

4. Group B Streptococcus (GBS) Screening: GBS screening is conducted late in pregnancy to identify if the mother is carrying the bacterium, which can be passed to the baby during childbirth.

5. Other Specialized Tests: Depending on the mother's medical history and risk factors, additional antenatal screening tests may be recommended, such as fetal echocardiography for heart abnormalities or amniocentesis for genetic testing.

Prenatal care and antenatal screening are essential for promoting the health of both the mother and the baby, detecting and managing any potential issues early, and ensuring a safe and successful pregnancy and delivery. Pregnant women should work closely with their healthcare providers to develop a personalized care plan that addresses their specific needs and circumstances.

High-Risk Pregnancy and Maternal Health

A high-risk pregnancy refers to a pregnancy in which the mother or the developing fetus has an increased chance of experiencing complications during pregnancy, childbirth, or postpartum. These complications can be related to pre-existing maternal health conditions, factors related to the pregnancy itself, or a combination of both. High-risk pregnancies require specialized medical care and monitoring to optimize maternal and fetal outcomes. Here are some factors that can contribute to a high-risk pregnancy and the importance of maternal health in such cases:

Factors Contributing to High-Risk Pregnancy:

1. Advanced Maternal Age: Pregnancy in women over the age of 35 is considered high-risk due to an increased risk of conditions like gestational diabetes, preeclampsia, and chromosomal abnormalities.
2. Pre-existing Medical Conditions: Women with pre-existing conditions such as diabetes, hypertension, heart disease, kidney disease, autoimmune disorders, and certain infections may have higher risks during pregnancy.
3. Multiple Pregnancies: Twin or higher-order multiple pregnancies are considered high-risk due to an increased chance of preterm birth and other complications.
4. Pregnancy-related Conditions: Conditions like gestational diabetes, preeclampsia (high blood pressure

during pregnancy), placenta previa (placenta covering the cervix), and placental abruption (premature detachment of the placenta) can pose risks to both the mother and the baby.

5. Previous Pregnancy Complications: Women who have experienced complications in previous pregnancies, such as preterm birth, recurrent miscarriages, or stillbirths, may have a higher risk of complications in subsequent pregnancies.

6. Lifestyle Factors: Smoking, alcohol consumption, drug use, and obesity can increase the risk of complications during pregnancy.

The Importance of Maternal Health in High-Risk Pregnancy:

1. Early Detection and Management: Early prenatal care is essential in identifying high-risk factors and medical conditions that may require specialized monitoring and management during pregnancy.

2. Regular Monitoring: Women with high-risk pregnancies require more frequent prenatal visits and specialized tests, such as ultrasounds and blood tests, to monitor the health of both the mother and the fetus.

3. Individualized Care Plan: Maternal health providers work with women with high-risk pregnancies to develop personalized care plans that address their specific needs and reduce the risk of complications.

4. Expert Medical Team: High-risk pregnancies are managed by a multidisciplinary team of healthcare providers, including obstetricians, maternal-fetal medicine specialists, neonatologists, and other specialists as needed.

5. Education and Support: Women with high-risk pregnancies and their families receive education about their condition, potential risks, and how to manage them effectively. Emotional support is also crucial in

navigating the challenges of a high-risk pregnancy.

6. Timely Interventions: In some cases, medical interventions, such as medications or specialized procedures, may be necessary to manage complications and optimize outcomes.

It's important for women with high-risk pregnancies to work closely with their healthcare providers, follow recommended guidelines, and prioritize their own health and well-being during pregnancy. Proper management and monitoring can significantly improve the chances of a successful pregnancy and the birth of a healthy baby.

Neonatal Care and the Neonatal Intensive Care Unit (NICU)

Neonatal care refers to specialized medical care provided to newborn infants, especially those born prematurely or with medical conditions that require close monitoring and treatment. Neonatal care is critical in ensuring the health and well-being of newborns during the early days and weeks of life. The Neonatal Intensive Care Unit (NICU) is a specialized unit within a hospital that provides intensive care to critically ill or premature newborns. Here's an overview of neonatal care and the NICU:

1. Neonatal Care:
   - Neonatal care begins immediately after birth and continues through the first weeks of life, especially for premature infants and those with medical conditions.
   - Newborns are assessed for vital signs, reflexes, weight, and any signs of distress or medical issues.
   - Basic neonatal care includes ensuring warmth, proper nutrition (breastfeeding or formula), and monitoring for signs of infection or other medical problems.

2. Neonatal Intensive Care Unit (NICU):
   - The NICU is a specialized unit in the hospital equipped with advanced medical equipment and staffed by healthcare professionals with expertise in neonatal care.
   - Infants admitted to the NICU may include

premature babies, those with respiratory distress, infections, congenital anomalies, or other critical medical conditions.

. The NICU provides constant monitoring of vital signs and specialized care tailored to each newborn's unique needs.

3. Services Provided in the NICU:

. Respiratory Support: Premature infants may need respiratory support such as mechanical ventilation or continuous positive airway pressure (CPAP) to assist with breathing.

. Temperature Regulation: Neonates are susceptible to heat loss, and the NICU ensures an appropriate warm environment for optimal growth and development.

. Feeding Support: For babies who cannot feed on their own, the NICU may provide nutrition through intravenous (IV) fluids or feeding tubes.

. Monitoring: Neonates in the NICU are continuously monitored for heart rate, breathing rate, oxygen saturation, and other vital signs.

. Medical Treatments: Infants in the NICU receive specialized medical treatments and medications as needed to manage specific conditions.

. Developmental Care: The NICU provides a developmentally supportive environment to promote the newborn's growth and neurodevelopment.

4. Family-Centered Care:

. NICUs aim to provide family-centered care, recognizing the importance of involving parents and supporting their emotional needs during their baby's stay in the unit.

- Parents are encouraged to participate in their baby's care, and education is provided to help them understand their infant's condition and treatment.

5. Gradual Transition:

- As newborns improve and stabilize, they may be gradually transitioned from the NICU to less intensive care settings within the hospital or transferred to a step-down nursery or special care nursery.

Neonatal care, particularly in the NICU, requires a highly specialized and dedicated team of healthcare professionals, including neonatologists, neonatal nurses, respiratory therapists, and other specialists. Their expertise and coordinated efforts are essential in providing the best possible care to newborns in critical situations. With advanced medical technology and skilled medical staff, many premature and critically ill newborns in the NICU can thrive and go on to lead healthy lives.

Common Neonatal Conditions and Prematurity

Common neonatal conditions and prematurity are significant factors that can impact the health and well-being of newborn infants. Prematurity refers to babies born before 37 weeks of gestation, while common neonatal conditions are health issues that may arise in newborns shortly after birth. Here are some common neonatal conditions and the impact of prematurity:

Common Neonatal Conditions:

1. Respiratory Distress Syndrome (RDS): RDS is a common condition in premature infants due to immature lung development. It can lead to breathing difficulties and requires respiratory support, such as surfactant administration and assisted ventilation.

2. Jaundice: Jaundice occurs when there is an excess of bilirubin in the blood, leading to yellowing of the skin and eyes. It is common in newborns and is usually mild and self-limiting, but severe cases may require phototherapy.

3. Sepsis: Newborns, especially premature infants, are at increased risk of developing sepsis, a severe bloodstream infection. Early recognition and prompt treatment with antibiotics are crucial to managing sepsis.

4. Hypoglycemia: Low blood sugar levels can occur in newborns, especially those born prematurely. Close monitoring and timely feeding or intravenous glucose administration may be required to manage

hypoglycemia.

5. Patent Ductus Arteriosus (PDA): PDA is a heart condition in which the ductus arteriosus, a blood vessel that bypasses the fetal lungs, remains open after birth. It can cause respiratory and circulatory problems and may require medical or surgical intervention.

6. Necrotizing Enterocolitis (NEC): NEC is a serious gastrointestinal condition that primarily affects premature infants. It involves inflammation and possible death of intestinal tissue and requires intensive medical management.

7. Intraventricular Hemorrhage (IVH): IVH is bleeding into the brain's ventricles and is more common in premature infants. The severity of IVH varies, and some cases resolve without long-term consequences.

Impact of Prematurity:

1. Respiratory Challenges: Premature babies often have immature lungs, making it challenging for them to breathe and maintain proper oxygen levels.

2. Temperature Instability: Premature infants have less body fat and struggle to regulate their body temperature, requiring a warm and controlled environment.

3. Immature Immune System: Premature babies have a less developed immune system, increasing their vulnerability to infections.

4. Feeding Difficulties: Premature infants may have difficulty breastfeeding or bottle-feeding due to weak sucking reflexes and poor coordination.

5. Neurodevelopmental Concerns: Premature birth is associated with an increased risk of neurodevelopmental issues, including cognitive and motor delays.

6. Growth and Weight Gain: Premature babies often

require special nutritional support to promote proper growth and weight gain.

With advances in medical care and technology, the outcomes for premature infants have improved significantly. Neonatal intensive care units (NICUs) provide specialized care and support to premature and critically ill newborns, giving them the best chance at a healthy start in life. Early and comprehensive neonatal care, along with ongoing monitoring and support, are essential to optimize the health and development of premature and medically fragile infants.

The First Days of Life: Newborn Care and Adaptation

The first days of life are a critical time for newborn care and adaptation as the baby transitions from the womb to the outside world. Newborns undergo significant changes as they adjust to their new environment, and proper care during this period is crucial for their health and well-being. Here are some key aspects of newborn care and adaptation during the first days of life:

1. Monitoring and Observation:
   - Newborns are closely monitored for vital signs, such as heart rate, respiratory rate, temperature, and blood oxygen levels, to ensure they are adapting well to life outside the womb.
   - Healthcare providers assess the baby's general appearance, reflexes, muscle tone, and behavior to check for any signs of distress or health issues.
2. Skin-to-Skin Contact:
   - Skin-to-skin contact, also known as kangaroo care, is encouraged immediately after birth and in the early days of life. This practice involves placing the baby on the mother's chest to promote bonding, regulate the baby's body temperature, and facilitate breastfeeding.
3. Feeding:
   - Breastfeeding is recommended as the best form of nutrition for newborns. In the first days of

life, babies may breastfeed frequently as they establish a feeding routine and stimulate milk production.
- For formula-fed infants, appropriate formula feeding practices are followed.

4. Cord Care:
- The baby's umbilical cord stump is kept clean and dry to prevent infection. It usually falls off within a few weeks.

5. Diapering and Hygiene:
- Newborns need frequent diaper changes to keep their skin clean and dry. Diapers should be changed promptly whenever wet or soiled.
- Bathing is typically delayed for a day or two after birth to allow the baby's natural skin barrier to develop fully.

6. Sleep and Wake Cycles:
- Newborns have irregular sleep patterns and may sleep for several hours at a time. It's essential to create a safe sleep environment and place the baby on their back to sleep to reduce the risk of sudden infant death syndrome (SIDS).

7. Neonatal Reflexes:
- Newborns have various reflexes, such as rooting (turning the head toward a touch on the cheek), grasping, and sucking, which are essential for feeding and interaction.

8. Jaundice Monitoring:
- Jaundice is common in newborns and typically appears a few days after birth. Healthcare providers monitor the baby's bilirubin levels and may recommend phototherapy if needed.

9. Family Bonding:
- Encouraging family bonding and involvement in newborn care is crucial for the baby's

emotional well-being and development.

10. Follow-Up Care:

- After hospital discharge, newborns may require follow-up visits with a pediatrician to ensure they are thriving and growing appropriately.

The first days of life are a precious time for parents and their newborns. Ensuring the baby's comfort, health, and safety through proper care and monitoring helps set the foundation for a positive start to life outside the womb. Regular communication with healthcare providers, asking questions, and seeking support as needed are essential for new parents to feel confident in caring for their newborn during this special time.

Breastfeeding and Infant Nutrition

Breastfeeding is the process of providing breast milk to infants for their nutrition and growth. It is widely recommended as the best source of nutrition for newborns and young infants due to its numerous health benefits. Breast milk is a unique and complete source of nutrition, specifically tailored to meet the needs of a growing baby. Here are some key aspects of breastfeeding and infant nutrition:

Benefits of Breastfeeding:

1. Optimal Nutrition: Breast milk provides all the essential nutrients, vitamins, and minerals necessary for a baby's growth and development during the first six months of life.
2. Immune Protection: Breast milk contains antibodies and other immune factors that help protect the baby from infections and illnesses, reducing the risk of respiratory and gastrointestinal infections.
3. Digestibility: Breast milk is easily digested by a baby's immature digestive system, leading to reduced instances of constipation and diarrhea.
4. Bonding and Emotional Health: Breastfeeding fosters bonding between the mother and baby and promotes emotional well-being for both.
5. Cognitive Development: Some studies suggest that breastfeeding may be associated with improved cognitive development in children.
6. Reduced Risk of Chronic Diseases: Breastfeeding has been linked to a reduced risk of obesity, type 2 diabetes, and certain allergic conditions later in life.

Breastfeeding Guidelines:

1. Exclusive Breastfeeding: The World Health Organization (WHO) and the American Academy of Pediatrics (AAP) recommend exclusive breastfeeding for the first six months of life. This means giving the baby only breast milk and no other food or drink, not even water, during this period.
2. Complementary Feeding: After six months, complementary foods can be introduced while continuing breastfeeding. Breastfeeding is encouraged until at least one year of age and beyond if mutually desired by the mother and baby.
3. On-Demand Feeding: Breastfed babies should be fed on-demand, which means allowing the baby to nurse whenever they show hunger cues, such as rooting, sucking on fists, or making sucking noises.
4. Proper Latch and Positioning: Correct latch and positioning are essential for effective breastfeeding and to prevent nipple discomfort or damage.
5. Avoidance of Formula Supplementation: To establish and maintain a good milk supply, it is generally recommended to avoid unnecessary formula supplementation in breastfed infants.

Infant Nutrition and Vitamin D:

- Breast milk provides most of the nutrients a baby needs, but the AAP recommends supplementing with vitamin D to ensure adequate intake, especially for exclusively breastfed infants.

Feeding Challenges and Support:

- Some mothers may face breastfeeding challenges, such as latching difficulties or concerns about milk supply. Seeking support from lactation consultants, healthcare providers, or breastfeeding support groups can be beneficial.

Breastfeeding is a personal choice, and while it is recommended for most infants, there are circumstances where formula feeding may be necessary or preferred. In such cases, commercial infant formulas provide appropriate nutrition for babies. The key is to provide adequate nutrition and loving care to support the healthy growth and development of the baby.

Infant Sleep and Caring for Sleep-Deprived Parents

Infant sleep patterns and caring for sleep-deprived parents are significant aspects of newborn care. Newborns have different sleep needs and patterns compared to older infants and adults. Sleep deprivation is common for parents of newborns, and finding ways to manage it effectively is crucial for their well-being and ability to care for their baby. Here are some key points about infant sleep and tips for caring for sleep-deprived parents:

Infant Sleep Patterns:

1. Sleep Duration: Newborns sleep for an average of 14 to 17 hours a day, but their sleep is typically fragmented into short periods, often lasting 2 to 4 hours at a time.
2. Day-Night Confusion: Newborns may have their days and nights mixed up initially, sleeping more during the day and being more wakeful at night. This can be challenging for parents trying to establish a sleep routine.
3. Frequent Night Waking: Newborns wake up frequently during the night to feed and fulfill their other needs, such as diaper changes and comfort.

Tips for Caring for Sleep-Deprived Parents:

1. Share Responsibilities: If possible, share nighttime responsibilities with a partner or other family members. Taking turns caring for the baby during the night can provide some relief to sleep-deprived parents.

2. Nap When the Baby Naps: Take advantage of the baby's daytime naps to catch up on sleep. Parents should prioritize rest and try to nap when the baby is sleeping.

3. Ask for Help: Reach out to friends and family for support. Accepting help with household chores or caring for the baby during the day can allow parents to get some much-needed rest.

4. Create a Soothing Sleep Environment: Establish a calming bedtime routine to help the baby transition to sleep at night. Creating a sleep-friendly environment with dim lighting and white noise may also help improve sleep for both the baby and parents.

5. Practice Safe Sleep: Follow safe sleep guidelines, such as placing the baby on their back to sleep, using a firm and flat sleep surface, and avoiding soft bedding or toys in the sleep area.

6. Seek Professional Support: If parents find themselves struggling with sleep deprivation or feelings of overwhelm, seeking support from a healthcare provider, counselor, or support group can be beneficial.

7. Prioritize Self-Care: It's essential for parents to take care of themselves physically and emotionally. Eating well, staying hydrated, and engaging in activities that promote relaxation and stress relief are important for overall well-being.

8. Be Patient and Flexible: Adjusting to a new sleep routine and caring for a newborn can be challenging. Parents should be patient with themselves and their baby during this time of adaptation.

Remember that newborn sleep patterns change as babies grow and develop. Over time, most infants gradually develop longer sleep stretches at night. However, sleep needs and patterns can vary from one baby to another. Being understanding, flexible, and responsive to the baby's needs can help parents navigate the challenges of sleep deprivation and create a nurturing and supportive environment for their newborn and themselves.

Infant Developmental Milestones

Infant developmental milestones are key achievements and skills that babies acquire as they grow and progress during the first year of life. Each milestone represents a significant step in the baby's physical, cognitive, and social development. It is important to remember that every baby is unique, and developmental milestones may be reached at slightly different ages. However, these are general guidelines for typical infant development:

1. Physical Development:
    - Head Control: By 3 to 4 months, babies can hold their head steady when supported in an upright position and can lift their head while lying on their tummy.
    - Rolling Over: Around 4 to 6 months, babies can roll over from tummy to back and back to tummy.
    - Sitting: By 6 to 8 months, babies can sit with support and, later on, without support.
    - Crawling and Mobility: Between 6 and 10 months, babies may begin to crawl or scoot on their belly and start pulling themselves up to stand.
    - Walking: Most babies take their first steps between 9 and 12 months, but the range can be broader.
2. Cognitive Development:
    - Social Smiles: Around 2 months, babies start to smile in response to familiar faces and voices.
    - Eye-Hand Coordination: By 3 to 4 months,

babies begin to reach for and grasp objects.

- Object Permanence: At around 6 to 9 months, babies develop an understanding that objects continue to exist even when they are out of sight.
- Babbling: Between 6 and 9 months, babies start to babble and imitate sounds and gestures.
- Cause and Effect: Around 9 to 12 months, babies begin to understand cause-and-effect relationships, such as pressing a button to make a toy produce sound.

3. Social and Emotional Development:
   - Attachment: Babies form strong emotional bonds with their primary caregivers from birth.
   - Social Interactions: Around 3 to 6 months, babies may begin to show interest in other people and engage in social interactions, such as smiling at others or cooing in response to voices.
   - Stranger Anxiety: Between 6 and 9 months, babies may start to show signs of anxiety or distress when encountering unfamiliar people.
   - Separation Anxiety: From around 9 months, babies may become upset when separated from their primary caregivers.

4. Communication and Language Development:
   - Cooing and Babbling: Between 2 and 6 months, babies start cooing and babbling, experimenting with different sounds.
   - Gestures: Around 8 to 12 months, babies may use gestures like pointing or waving to communicate.
   - First Words: By 9 to 12 months, some babies may say their first words, typically simple syllables like "mama" or "dada."

Remember that each baby develops at their own pace, and there is a wide range of normal development. If you have concerns about your baby's development or if they seem to be significantly delayed in reaching milestones, it's essential to discuss your observations with a pediatrician or healthcare provider for further evaluation and guidance.

Nutritional Needs of Infants, Toddlers, and Children

The nutritional needs of infants, toddlers, and children differ at each stage of their development. Providing age-appropriate and balanced nutrition is crucial for supporting growth, development, and overall health. Here are the nutritional needs for each age group:

1. Infants (0-12 months):
   - Breast Milk or Formula: Breast milk or infant formula is the primary source of nutrition for infants up to 6 months of age. It provides essential nutrients, antibodies, and promotes optimal growth and development.
   - Introduction of Solid Foods: Starting around 6 months, complementary solid foods are gradually introduced while continuing breast milk or formula. Iron-fortified cereals, pureed fruits and vegetables, and age-appropriate protein sources (e.g., pureed meats, beans, and tofu) are introduced.
2. Toddlers (1-3 years):
   - Balanced Diet: Toddlers need a balanced diet that includes a variety of foods from all food groups, such as fruits, vegetables, whole grains, proteins (e.g., meat, fish, poultry, eggs, legumes), and dairy products or dairy alternatives.
   - Healthy Fats: Healthy fats are essential for

brain development. Sources include avocados, nuts, seeds, and oils like olive oil.

- Limited Added Sugars and Salt: Minimize added sugars and salt in the toddler's diet to foster healthy eating habits.

3. Preschoolers and Young Children (4-8 years):
   - Variety of Foods: Encourage a wide variety of foods to meet nutritional needs and expose children to different flavors and textures.
   - Calcium-Rich Foods: Dairy products, fortified plant-based milk, and leafy green vegetables are good sources of calcium for bone health.
   - Iron-Rich Foods: Iron-rich foods, such as lean meats, beans, and fortified cereals, are important for cognitive development and energy.

4. School-Age Children (9-13 years) and Adolescents (14-18 years):
   - Nutrient-Dense Foods: Emphasize nutrient-dense foods that provide essential vitamins and minerals without excessive calories.
   - Hydration: Encourage drinking water and limiting sugary beverages.
   - Balanced Meals: Meals should include a mix of carbohydrates, proteins, healthy fats, and plenty of fruits and vegetables.

It's essential to encourage healthy eating habits from an early age, as these habits can influence a child's lifelong eating patterns and overall health. Here are some general tips for promoting healthy eating in children:

- Lead by Example: Demonstrate healthy eating habits yourself, as children often model their behavior after adults.
- Family Meals: Eating together as a family promotes

positive associations with mealtimes and encourages healthier food choices.

- Limit Processed Foods: Reduce the consumption of processed and sugary foods and opt for whole, natural foods whenever possible.
- Be Patient: Children may be selective eaters or go through phases of food preferences. Be patient and offer a variety of nutritious options.

Always consult with a pediatrician or registered dietitian to address specific dietary needs and ensure that children are meeting their nutritional requirements at each stage of development.

Healthy Eating Habits for Children

Promoting healthy eating habits in children is essential for their growth, development, and overall well-being. Establishing positive eating behaviors from an early age can set the foundation for a lifetime of healthy choices. Here are some tips to encourage healthy eating habits for children:

1. Offer a Variety of Nutritious Foods:
   - Provide a wide range of foods from all food groups, including fruits, vegetables, whole grains, lean proteins, and dairy products or dairy alternatives.
   - Introduce new foods gradually and repeatedly, as it may take several exposures for children to accept and enjoy new flavors.
2. Be a Role Model:
   - Children learn by example, so demonstrate healthy eating habits yourself. Eat a balanced diet and show enthusiasm for trying new foods.
3. Eat Together as a Family:
   - Family meals provide an opportunity for connection and positive associations with healthy foods. Aim to eat together as a family as often as possible.
4. Avoid Restrictive Diets:
   - Avoid putting children on strict diets or labeling foods as "good" or "bad." Instead, focus on balance and moderation in food choices.
5. Limit Sugary and Processed Foods:

- Minimize the consumption of sugary snacks, candies, sugary beverages, and processed foods high in added sugars and unhealthy fats.

6. Encourage Water Consumption:
   - Offer water as the primary beverage for thirst and hydration, rather than sugary drinks.

7. Involve Children in Meal Planning and Preparation:
   - Let children help with grocery shopping, meal planning, and food preparation. Involving them in these activities can increase their interest in trying new foods.

8. Offer Healthy Snacks:
   - Have a variety of healthy snacks readily available, such as cut fruits, vegetables, yogurt, whole-grain crackers, and nuts.

9. Be Patient with Picky Eating:
   - Picky eating is common in young children. Offer a balanced meal and allow them to choose from the options provided. Avoid pressuring or forcing them to eat specific foods.

10. Practice Mindful Eating:
   - Encourage mindful eating by slowing down during meals, savoring the flavors, and paying attention to hunger and fullness cues.

11. Limit Screen Time during Meals:
   - Create a screen-free zone during mealtime to promote family interaction and focus on eating.

12. Celebrate Food and Cultural Diversity:
   - Teach children about different cuisines and celebrate cultural diversity through food exploration.

13. Use Positive Reinforcement:
   - Praise and encourage children when they make healthy food choices, but avoid using food as a reward.

Remember that developing healthy eating habits is a gradual process. Be patient, flexible, and supportive in encouraging children to make nutritious choices. Consistency and a positive food environment at home can significantly impact children's attitudes towards food and healthy eating throughout their lives. If you have concerns about your child's eating habits or nutrition, consider consulting with a pediatrician or a registered dietitian for personalized guidance.

Managing Picky Eaters and Food Allergies

Managing picky eaters and food allergies can be challenging for parents and caregivers. Both situations require a thoughtful and individualized approach to ensure that children receive adequate nutrition and have a positive relationship with food. Here are some strategies for managing picky eaters and handling food allergies:

Managing Picky Eaters:

1. Be Patient and Persistent:
    - Picky eating is common in young children, and it may take several attempts before they accept new foods. Continue offering a variety of nutritious options and be patient with their preferences.
2. Offer a Balanced Diet:
    - Even if a child is selective about certain foods, make sure to provide a balanced diet with a variety of fruits, vegetables, whole grains, proteins, and dairy or dairy alternatives.
3. Involve Children in Meal Planning and Preparation:
    - Let children help choose foods at the grocery store and involve them in age-appropriate meal preparation. This can increase their interest in trying new foods.
4. Make Meals Fun and Colorful:
    - Present food in a visually appealing way and

use fun plates, cups, and utensils. Experiment with different shapes and colors to make meals more enticing.

5. Offer Dips and Sauces:
   - Dips like hummus, yogurt, or nut butter can make vegetables and other foods more enjoyable for picky eaters.

6. Avoid Pressure and Power Struggles:
   - Pressuring or forcing a child to eat specific foods can create negative associations with mealtimes. Instead, offer a variety of choices and let them decide what and how much to eat.

Handling Food Allergies:

1. Identify Allergens:
   - If a child has been diagnosed with a food allergy, it is essential to identify and eliminate the allergenic food from their diet. Common allergens include milk, eggs, peanuts, tree nuts, soy, wheat, fish, and shellfish.

2. Read Food Labels Carefully:
   - Learn to read food labels to identify potential allergens in packaged foods. Look for hidden ingredients and cross-contamination risks.

3. Inform Caregivers and Schools:
   - Inform caregivers, teachers, and school staff about the child's food allergy. Ensure that they understand the severity of the allergy and know how to respond in case of an allergic reaction.

4. Create a Safe Food Environment:
   - Keep allergenic foods out of the child's reach and ensure that food preparation areas are thoroughly cleaned to prevent cross-contamination.

5. Always Carry Medications:
  - If prescribed by a doctor, ensure that the child carries their epinephrine auto-injector (e.g., EpiPen) at all times in case of accidental exposure.
6. Offer Safe Alternatives:
  - Find safe and nutritious alternatives to replace allergenic foods in the child's diet.
7. Teach Self-Advocacy:
  - As the child gets older, teach them to be aware of their allergies and how to communicate their needs to others.

Seeking guidance from a pediatrician or a registered dietitian can be helpful when managing picky eating or food allergies. They can provide personalized advice and address any specific concerns related to the child's health and dietary needs. Patience, understanding, and support are essential in both situations to ensure the child's well-being and promote a positive and healthy relationship with food.

Cognitive, Social, and Emotional Development

Cognitive, social, and emotional development are interconnected aspects of a child's growth and maturation. Each domain plays a crucial role in shaping a child's overall development and abilities. Here's an overview of each area:

1. Cognitive Development:
   - Cognitive development refers to the growth and improvement of a child's mental processes, including thinking, learning, problem-solving, memory, and understanding of the world around them.
   - Piaget's stages of cognitive development provide a framework for understanding how children's thinking evolves from infancy through adolescence. These stages include sensorimotor, preoperational, concrete operational, and formal operational stages.
   - Key milestones in cognitive development include object permanence (understanding that objects exist even when not visible), symbolic play, language development, and logical reasoning.
2. Social Development:
   - Social development involves a child's interactions with others and the development of social skills, relationships, and understanding of social norms and roles.

- During infancy, social development includes forming attachments to caregivers and developing social smiles and communication through gestures and cooing.
- In early childhood, children start to engage in parallel play (playing alongside but not with other children) and gradually progress to cooperative play (playing together and sharing with others).
- Social development also includes the development of empathy, understanding others' emotions, and recognizing social cues such as facial expressions and body language.

3. Emotional Development:
   - Emotional development refers to the growth and understanding of a child's emotions, as well as their ability to manage and express emotions appropriately.
   - In infancy, emotions are more basic, such as joy, sadness, and distress. As children grow, they begin to experience a broader range of emotions, including empathy, jealousy, pride, and guilt.
   - Emotional development involves learning to identify and label emotions, understand the causes of emotions, and develop strategies to regulate emotions effectively.

Interplay of Domains:

- Cognitive, social, and emotional development are interconnected and mutually influence each other. For example, social interactions can stimulate cognitive development, and emotional experiences can impact social relationships.
- The development of a strong emotional foundation

supports social relationships and the ability to form positive connections with others.

- Cognitive skills, such as problem-solving and perspective-taking, contribute to social interactions and emotional understanding.

Promoting Healthy Development:

- Providing a nurturing and responsive environment that supports cognitive, social, and emotional growth is essential for a child's healthy development.
- Engaging in activities that stimulate cognitive skills, encouraging positive social interactions and play, and fostering emotional expression and regulation are all important for supporting development in these domains.
- Responsive caregiving, active listening, and validating a child's feelings can nurture emotional well-being and healthy social interactions.

Overall, cognitive, social, and emotional development are intricately connected and contribute to a child's overall growth and functioning. Supporting each domain and recognizing the importance of their interactions can help children thrive and reach their full potential.

Behavioral Challenges and Discipline Strategies

Behavioral challenges are common in children as they grow and develop. Understanding age-appropriate behaviors and employing effective discipline strategies are essential for promoting positive behavior and managing challenging situations. Here are some tips for addressing behavioral challenges and implementing discipline strategies:

1. Understand Developmental Stages:
   - Recognize that age and developmental stages play a significant role in a child's behavior. What may be considered challenging behavior at one age might be developmentally appropriate at another.
2. Set Clear Expectations:
   - Establish clear and age-appropriate expectations for behavior. Communicate these expectations consistently to the child.
3. Positive Reinforcement:
   - Use positive reinforcement, praise, and encouragement to acknowledge and reward good behavior. Positive reinforcement can motivate children to repeat positive behaviors.
4. Consistency:
   - Consistency is key in discipline. Be consistent in enforcing rules and consequences to help children understand the expected behavior.
5. Time-In and Time-Out:

- For younger children, time-in (spending time with the caregiver to talk and calm down) can be more effective than traditional time-outs. Time-outs can be used for older children when they need a brief break to regain self-control.

6. Redirecting Behavior:
    - For minor misbehaviors, redirect the child's attention to a different activity or area to shift their focus.

7. Use "I" Statements:
    - Use "I" statements to express your feelings and expectations, such as "I feel upset when toys are not put away."

8. Avoid Physical Punishment:
    - Avoid physical punishment, as it can harm the child's emotional well-being and lead to negative outcomes.

9. Time and Space for Calm Discussions:
    - Allow time and space for calm discussions about behavior and consequences. Discuss the reasons behind rules and encourage the child to express their feelings.

10. Teach Problem-Solving Skills:
    - Help children develop problem-solving skills to deal with conflicts and challenges in a constructive manner.

11. Model Appropriate Behavior:
    - Be a positive role model for the behavior you want to see in your child. Children often learn by observing their caregivers.

12. Use Natural Consequences:
    - Allow children to experience natural consequences of their actions whenever appropriate. Natural consequences are the direct result of a child's behavior (e.g., not wearing a jacket results in feeling cold).

13. Communicate with Empathy:

- Communicate with empathy and understanding when addressing behavioral challenges. Recognize and acknowledge the child's feelings while also guiding them toward appropriate behavior.

It's important to remember that discipline is about teaching and guiding children rather than punishing them. Creating a positive and supportive environment, fostering open communication, and recognizing children's individual needs can contribute to successful discipline and the development of positive behavior patterns. For more challenging behaviors or persistent concerns, consider seeking guidance from a pediatrician, child psychologist, or parenting support group.

Autism Spectrum Disorder and Developmental Delays

Autism Spectrum Disorder (ASD) and developmental delays are two distinct but related concepts that affect a child's development and behavior. Let's understand each term separately:

1. Autism Spectrum Disorder (ASD):
    - ASD is a neurodevelopmental disorder that affects communication, social interaction, and behavior. It is characterized by a wide range of symptoms and challenges that can vary significantly from one person to another.
    - Common symptoms of ASD include difficulties in social communication and interaction, repetitive behaviors, restricted interests, and sensory sensitivities.
    - ASD is referred to as a "spectrum" because individuals with the condition can have varying degrees of impairment and strengths in different areas.
    - Early signs of ASD may appear in infancy or early childhood, and a diagnosis is typically made based on behavioral observations and assessments.

2. Developmental Delays:
    - Developmental delays refer to significant delays or lags in achieving age-appropriate milestones across various areas of development, including physical, cognitive,

communication, social, and emotional skills.

- Developmental delays can be caused by a variety of factors, including genetic conditions, prematurity, neurological disorders, or environmental factors.
- Early intervention and appropriate support can be beneficial in addressing developmental delays and promoting healthy development.

Relation between ASD and Developmental Delays:

- Developmental delays can be a feature of ASD, as many individuals with ASD may have delays in reaching certain developmental milestones.
- However, not all children with developmental delays have ASD. Delays can be caused by various factors, and some children may have delays in specific areas while developing typically in others.
- ASD is diagnosed based on specific criteria outlined in the Diagnostic and Statistical Manual of Mental Disorders (DSM-5). It is a comprehensive evaluation that considers communication, social behavior, repetitive behaviors, and other associated features.

Early Identification and Intervention:

- Early identification and intervention are crucial for children with developmental delays and ASD.
- Early intervention services, such as speech therapy, occupational therapy, behavioral therapy, and special education, can help address developmental challenges and support the child's progress.
- If parents or caregivers have concerns about their child's development, it is essential to seek evaluation and guidance from healthcare professionals and specialists.

Every child is unique, and early identification and support can significantly impact a child's development and long-term outcomes. The goal is to provide tailored interventions and support that address the child's specific needs, strengths, and challenges to help them reach their full potential.

Pediatric Cardiology: Heart Health in Children

Pediatric cardiology is a specialized branch of medicine that focuses on the diagnosis and treatment of heart conditions in children, including newborns, infants, children, and adolescents. Heart health in children is essential for their overall well-being and proper growth and development. Here are some key aspects of pediatric cardiology and heart health in children:

1. Congenital Heart Defects (CHDs):
   - Congenital heart defects are structural abnormalities of the heart that are present at birth. They can range from mild to severe and may affect the heart's chambers, valves, or major blood vessels.
   - Early detection and appropriate management of CHDs are crucial for the best possible outcomes. Many CHDs can be diagnosed before or shortly after birth through prenatal screenings or newborn screenings.
2. Acquired Heart Conditions:
   - Children can also develop acquired heart conditions, such as myocarditis (inflammation of the heart muscle), Kawasaki disease (an inflammatory condition affecting blood vessels), and arrhythmias (abnormal heart rhythms).
   - Timely diagnosis and treatment of acquired heart conditions are essential to prevent

complications and promote recovery.

3. Heart Murmurs:
   - Heart murmurs are abnormal sounds heard during a heartbeat and are common in children. Not all heart murmurs indicate a heart problem, but they should be evaluated by a pediatric cardiologist to determine their cause and significance.

4. Screening and Diagnostic Tests:
   - Pediatric cardiologists use various screening and diagnostic tests, such as echocardiograms, electrocardiograms (ECGs or EKGs), and cardiac catheterization, to evaluate heart health and diagnose heart conditions in children.

5. Heart Health Promotion:
   - Promoting heart health in children includes advocating for a healthy lifestyle, including a balanced diet, regular physical activity, and maintaining a healthy weight.
   - Avoiding exposure to tobacco smoke and promoting a smoke-free environment is essential for heart health in children and can reduce the risk of heart disease later in life.

6. Prevention of Rheumatic Heart Disease (RHD):
   - Rheumatic heart disease is a preventable condition that results from untreated strep throat infections. Timely treatment of strep throat with antibiotics can prevent RHD.

7. Cardiac Rehabilitation:
   - For children with complex heart conditions or those who have undergone heart surgery, cardiac rehabilitation programs may be recommended to support their recovery and improve their overall heart health.

8. Long-Term Follow-Up:
   - Children with heart conditions require regular

follow-up with a pediatric cardiologist to monitor their heart health, manage any ongoing issues, and adjust treatment as needed.

It's essential for parents and caregivers to be vigilant about their child's heart health and to seek prompt medical attention if they notice any signs or symptoms of heart problems. Early detection, proper diagnosis, and appropriate management of heart conditions in children can significantly improve outcomes and enhance their quality of life. Pediatric cardiologists play a vital role in the comprehensive care of children with heart conditions, providing specialized expertise and guidance for their heart health journey.

Pediatric Pulmonology: Respiratory Health in Children

Pediatric pulmonology is a medical specialty that focuses on the respiratory health of children, from newborns to adolescents. Pediatric pulmonologists are experts in diagnosing and treating a wide range of respiratory conditions and disorders that affect the lungs and airways in children. Here are some key aspects of pediatric pulmonology and respiratory health in children:

1. Common Respiratory Conditions:
   - Pediatric pulmonologists diagnose and manage various respiratory conditions, including asthma, bronchitis, pneumonia, bronchiolitis, cystic fibrosis, congenital lung abnormalities, and chronic cough.
2. Asthma:
   - Asthma is a chronic condition characterized by inflammation and narrowing of the airways, leading to breathing difficulties, wheezing, and coughing.
   - Pediatric pulmonologists work with children and their families to develop personalized asthma action plans to manage symptoms and prevent asthma attacks.
3. Bronchitis and Pneumonia:
   - Bronchitis is inflammation of the bronchial tubes, and pneumonia is an infection that causes inflammation in the air sacs of the lungs.

- Pediatric pulmonologists provide treatment to help resolve the infection and support lung healing.

4. Bronchiolitis:
    - Bronchiolitis is a common respiratory infection in young children, usually caused by a viral infection that affects the small airways in the lungs.
    - Treatment may include supportive care, such as maintaining hydration and providing supplemental oxygen if needed.

5. Cystic Fibrosis (CF):
    - Cystic fibrosis is a genetic disorder that affects the lungs and digestive system, causing thick, sticky mucus to build up in the airways.
    - Pediatric pulmonologists work with a multidisciplinary team to manage CF and improve lung function and overall health.

6. Sleep-Related Breathing Disorders:
    - Pediatric pulmonologists evaluate and treat sleep-related breathing disorders, such as sleep apnea and snoring, which can affect a child's quality of sleep and overall health.

7. Lung Function Testing:
    - Pulmonary function tests are commonly used to assess lung function and help diagnose and manage respiratory conditions in children.

8. Allergy and Immunology:
    - Some pediatric pulmonologists may also have expertise in allergy and immunology, as allergies can significantly impact respiratory health.

9. Long-Term Management and Follow-Up:
    - Pediatric pulmonologists work closely with children and their families to provide ongoing management and follow-up care for chronic

respiratory conditions.

10. Prevention and Education:

- Pediatric pulmonologists play a role in educating families about preventive measures to reduce the risk of respiratory infections and manage chronic conditions effectively.

Maintaining respiratory health in children involves early detection, timely treatment, and a comprehensive approach to care. Regular check-ups with a pediatric pulmonologist are essential for children with respiratory conditions to monitor lung function, adjust treatment plans, and optimize overall respiratory health. Parents and caregivers should seek medical attention promptly if they notice any signs or symptoms of respiratory problems in their children.

Pediatric Neurology: Brain and Nervous System Health

Pediatric neurology is a medical specialty that focuses on the diagnosis and management of disorders related to the brain, spinal cord, peripheral nerves, and muscles in children and adolescents. Pediatric neurologists are specialized doctors who have expertise in treating a wide range of neurological conditions in children. Here are some key aspects of pediatric neurology and brain and nervous system health in children:

1. Neurological Disorders in Children:
    - Pediatric neurologists diagnose and treat various neurological disorders, including epilepsy and seizure disorders, headaches and migraines, developmental delays, cerebral palsy, neuromuscular disorders, neurogenetic disorders, and neurodevelopmental disorders (e.g., autism spectrum disorder).
2. Epilepsy and Seizure Disorders:
    - Epilepsy is a common neurological condition characterized by recurrent seizures. Pediatric neurologists work to diagnose the type of seizures and provide appropriate treatment, such as anti-seizure medications or other therapies.
3. Developmental Delays and Neurodevelopmental Disorders:
    - Pediatric neurologists play a role in evaluating and managing developmental delays, which

may be related to neurological issues. They also work with other specialists to diagnose and support children with neurodevelopmental disorders like autism spectrum disorder.

4. Cerebral Palsy:
   - Cerebral palsy is a group of movement disorders caused by brain damage that occurs before, during, or shortly after birth. Pediatric neurologists work to manage and support children with cerebral palsy to optimize their function and quality of life.

5. Headaches and Migraines:
   - Pediatric neurologists assess and treat headaches and migraines in children, which can significantly impact a child's daily life and well-being.

6. Neuromuscular Disorders:
   - Pediatric neurologists diagnose and manage neuromuscular disorders that affect the muscles and nerves, such as muscular dystrophy and myasthenia gravis.

7. Neurogenetic Disorders:
   - Pediatric neurologists are involved in diagnosing and managing neurogenetic disorders, which are conditions caused by genetic abnormalities affecting the nervous system.

8. Neuroimaging and Diagnostic Testing:
   - Neuroimaging, such as MRI and CT scans, and other diagnostic tests are used by pediatric neurologists to assess brain and nervous system health and aid in the diagnosis of neurological conditions.

9. Treatment Planning and Management:
   - Pediatric neurologists work with a multidisciplinary team to develop

individualized treatment plans for each child based on their specific neurological condition and needs.

10. Support and Education:
   - Pediatric neurologists provide support and education to families, empowering them to understand their child's condition and actively participate in their care.

Maintaining brain and nervous system health is crucial for children's overall well-being and development. Early detection, prompt intervention, and ongoing management are essential in pediatric neurology to optimize outcomes and improve the quality of life for children with neurological disorders. Parents and caregivers should seek medical attention if they notice any signs or symptoms of neurological issues in their children, such as seizures, developmental delays, motor difficulties, or changes in behavior.

Pediatric Gastroenterology: Digestive Health in Children

Pediatric gastroenterology is a medical specialty that focuses on the diagnosis and treatment of disorders related to the digestive system in children and adolescents. Pediatric gastroenterologists are specialized doctors who have expertise in addressing a wide range of gastrointestinal (GI) and nutritional issues in children. Here are some key aspects of pediatric gastroenterology and digestive health in children:

1. Common Digestive Disorders:
   - Pediatric gastroenterologists diagnose and manage various digestive disorders, including gastroesophageal reflux disease (GERD), inflammatory bowel disease (IBD), celiac disease, constipation, diarrhea, food allergies, and more.

2. Gastroesophageal Reflux Disease (GERD):
   - GERD is a condition in which stomach acid flows back into the esophagus, causing symptoms such as heartburn and regurgitation. Pediatric gastroenterologists provide treatment and guidance for managing GERD in children.

3. Inflammatory Bowel Disease (IBD):
   - IBD includes conditions like Crohn's disease and ulcerative colitis, which cause chronic inflammation in the digestive tract. Pediatric gastroenterologists work to diagnose and

manage IBD and improve quality of life for affected children.

4. Celiac Disease:
   - Celiac disease is an autoimmune disorder in which the ingestion of gluten triggers an immune response that damages the small intestine. Pediatric gastroenterologists diagnose and guide children and their families in managing a gluten-free diet.

5. Food Allergies and Intolerances:
   - Pediatric gastroenterologists diagnose and manage food allergies, sensitivities, and intolerances that can affect the digestive system and overall health.

6. Nutritional Assessment and Support:
   - Pediatric gastroenterologists assess and address nutritional issues, such as poor weight gain, growth concerns, and feeding difficulties in children.

7. Diagnostic Procedures:
   - Pediatric gastroenterologists use various diagnostic procedures, such as endoscopy, colonoscopy, and imaging studies, to evaluate the GI tract and identify underlying issues.

8. Support for Children with Complex Conditions:
   - Pediatric gastroenterologists work with children who have complex medical conditions, such as congenital anomalies, motility disorders, and gastrointestinal complications of other systemic conditions.

9. Long-Term Management and Follow-Up:
   - Pediatric gastroenterologists provide ongoing care and follow-up for children with chronic digestive conditions to monitor progress and adjust treatment plans as needed.

10. Nutritional Guidance:

- Pediatric gastroenterologists collaborate with registered dietitians to provide nutritional guidance and dietary recommendations tailored to each child's specific needs.

Digestive health is vital for children's overall well-being, growth, and development. Parents and caregivers should seek medical attention if they notice any signs or symptoms of digestive issues in their children, such as persistent abdominal pain, vomiting, diarrhea, or changes in bowel habits. Pediatric gastroenterologists play a critical role in diagnosing and managing digestive disorders in children and improving their quality of life.

Pediatric Oncology: Childhood Cancer Care

Pediatric oncology is a specialized medical field that focuses on the diagnosis, treatment, and care of children and adolescents with cancer. Childhood cancer is different from adult cancer and requires a multidisciplinary approach involving pediatric oncologists, surgeons, radiation oncologists, nurses, social workers, and other healthcare professionals. Here are some key aspects of pediatric oncology and childhood cancer care:

1. Types of Childhood Cancers:
   - Childhood cancers differ from adult cancers in terms of the types of tumors and their treatment approaches. Common childhood cancers include leukemia, brain tumors, neuroblastoma, Wilms tumor, lymphoma, and bone tumors.

2. Early Diagnosis and Staging:
   - Early diagnosis is crucial in childhood cancer to ensure timely treatment and improved outcomes. Accurate staging determines the extent of the disease and guides treatment decisions.

3. Multidisciplinary Care:
   - Pediatric oncology teams consist of various specialists who collaborate to develop comprehensive treatment plans that address the unique needs of each child. Treatment plans often include a combination of surgery,

chemotherapy, radiation therapy, and targeted therapies.

4. Supportive Care:
   - Supportive care is an integral part of pediatric oncology and focuses on managing side effects of treatments, providing pain management, addressing emotional and psychological needs, and enhancing the overall well-being of the child and their family.

5. Pediatric Oncology Research:
   - Ongoing research in pediatric oncology aims to improve treatment outcomes and quality of life for children with cancer. Clinical trials are often conducted to evaluate new treatments and therapies.

6. Survivorship:
   - Advances in treatment have led to increased survival rates for many childhood cancers. Pediatric oncologists provide long-term follow-up care for survivors, addressing potential late effects of treatment and ensuring their overall health.

7. Psychosocial Support:
   - Childhood cancer affects the emotional well-being of both the child and their family. Psychosocial support services, including counseling, support groups, and art therapy, help children and families cope with the challenges of cancer.

8. Palliative and Hospice Care:
   - In cases where a cure is not possible, pediatric oncology teams provide palliative care to manage symptoms and improve the child's comfort and quality of life. Hospice care offers support to families during the end-of-life journey.

9. Family-Centered Care:
   - Pediatric oncology emphasizes family-centered care, involving parents and caregivers in treatment decisions and providing emotional and practical support throughout the cancer journey.

Childhood cancer is a complex and challenging medical condition, and the care provided by pediatric oncologists and the multidisciplinary team is essential for the best possible outcomes. Families facing childhood cancer should work closely with their pediatric oncology team to understand treatment options, make informed decisions, and receive comprehensive support throughout the entire process.

Childhood Diabetes and Endocrine Disorders

Childhood diabetes and endocrine disorders refer to a group of medical conditions that affect the endocrine system, which is responsible for producing hormones that regulate various bodily functions. Two common conditions within this group are childhood diabetes, specifically type 1 diabetes, and various endocrine disorders that can affect growth, metabolism, and hormonal balance in children. Here's an overview of childhood diabetes and endocrine disorders:

1. Childhood Diabetes (Type 1 Diabetes):
    - Type 1 diabetes is an autoimmune condition in which the body's immune system mistakenly attacks and destroys the insulin-producing cells in the pancreas. Insulin is a hormone that regulates blood sugar levels.
    - Symptoms of type 1 diabetes in children include excessive thirst, frequent urination, weight loss, increased hunger, fatigue, and blurry vision.
    - Management of type 1 diabetes involves daily insulin injections or the use of an insulin pump to maintain stable blood sugar levels. Monitoring blood sugar levels, adhering to a balanced diet, and regular physical activity are also important components of diabetes management.
    - Pediatric endocrinologists play a key role in

diagnosing and managing type 1 diabetes in children, providing guidance on insulin administration, monitoring, and dietary management.

2. Endocrine Disorders Affecting Growth and Development:
   - Pediatric endocrinologists diagnose and treat various endocrine disorders that affect growth and development, such as growth hormone deficiency, precocious puberty (early puberty), and delayed puberty.
   - Growth hormone deficiency can be treated with synthetic growth hormone to promote normal growth in children who have insufficient levels of the hormone.

3. Thyroid Disorders:
   - Pediatric endocrinologists manage thyroid disorders in children, including hypothyroidism (underactive thyroid) and hyperthyroidism (overactive thyroid). These conditions can affect metabolism, energy levels, and overall health.

4. Adrenal Disorders:
   - Adrenal disorders, such as congenital adrenal hyperplasia or adrenal insufficiency, involve the dysfunction of the adrenal glands and can impact hormone production and regulation.

5. Metabolic Disorders:
   - Some endocrine disorders are related to metabolism, such as disorders of glucose metabolism, lipid metabolism, and calcium metabolism. These conditions can have a significant impact on overall health and require specialized care.

6. Pituitary Disorders:
   - Disorders affecting the pituitary gland can

lead to hormonal imbalances and affect growth, reproduction, and other bodily functions. Pediatric endocrinologists diagnose and manage these conditions.

7. Multidisciplinary Care:
   - Children with diabetes and endocrine disorders often require multidisciplinary care involving pediatric endocrinologists, registered dietitians, nurses, social workers, and other healthcare professionals.

Early diagnosis, appropriate treatment, and regular follow-up are crucial for managing childhood diabetes and endocrine disorders. Pediatric endocrinologists play a vital role in providing specialized care, guidance, and support to children and their families. Parents and caregivers should seek medical attention if they notice any signs or symptoms of diabetes or endocrine disorders in their children, such as changes in growth, development, or energy levels.

Managing Chronic Conditions in Children

Managing chronic conditions in children requires a comprehensive and coordinated approach that addresses the physical, emotional, social, and psychological aspects of the child's health. Chronic conditions can include conditions like asthma, diabetes, epilepsy, cystic fibrosis, autoimmune disorders, and more. Here are some key strategies for managing chronic conditions in children effectively:

1. Develop a Strong Care Team:
   - Build a care team that includes healthcare professionals with expertise in the specific chronic condition, such as pediatricians, specialists, nurses, dietitians, therapists, and social workers.
2. Educate Yourself and Your Child:
   - Gain a thorough understanding of the chronic condition, its management, treatment options, and potential complications. Educate your child in age-appropriate ways so they can be actively involved in their care.
3. Establish a Care Plan:
   - Work with your healthcare team to develop a personalized care plan that outlines medication schedules, treatment goals, dietary recommendations, and strategies for managing symptoms.
4. Regular Medical Checkups:
   - Schedule regular follow-up appointments with your child's healthcare provider to monitor

their condition, adjust treatments as needed, and address any concerns.

5. Medication Management:

   · Ensure that medications are taken as prescribed. Teach your child the importance of medication adherence and involve them in managing their medications as they grow older.

6. Monitoring and Self-Care:

   · Teach your child to monitor their symptoms, track key indicators (such as blood sugar levels), and practice self-care routines as appropriate. Encourage them to communicate any changes to the care team.

7. Lifestyle Management:

   · Help your child adopt a healthy lifestyle that includes a balanced diet, regular exercise, adequate sleep, and stress reduction. These factors can positively impact overall health and condition management.

8. Emotional Support:

   · Children with chronic conditions may experience emotional challenges. Offer emotional support, encourage open communication, and consider involving a therapist or counselor to help them cope.

9. School and Social Activities:

   · Collaborate with teachers, school staff, and other caregivers to ensure that your child's needs are met at school. Encourage your child to participate in social activities while also managing their condition.

10. Advocacy:

   · Be an advocate for your child's health needs. Work with the care team to ensure that the child's rights and well-being are upheld in all settings.

11. Transition to Adulthood:

- As your child grows, gradually involve them in managing their own care. Help them transition to adult healthcare providers and support them in taking ownership of their health.

12. Community Resources and Support Groups:

- Connect with local and online support groups for families facing similar challenges. These groups can provide valuable advice, resources, and a sense of community.

Managing a chronic condition in a child requires ongoing effort, communication, and a collaborative approach between the child, caregivers, and healthcare professionals. By working together, families can help children lead fulfilling lives while effectively managing their health conditions.

Supporting Families of Children with Chronic Illnesses

Supporting families of children with chronic illnesses is essential for helping them navigate the challenges that come with managing their child's health condition. Chronic illnesses can have a significant impact on the child and the entire family, both emotionally and practically. Here are ways to provide support to families facing this situation:

1. Empathy and Understanding:
   - Show empathy and understanding towards the challenges the family is facing. Acknowledge their feelings and offer a listening ear.
2. Educate and Inform:
   - Provide accurate and clear information about the child's condition, treatment options, and management strategies. Empower families to make informed decisions.
3. Multidisciplinary Care:
   - Involve a multidisciplinary team of healthcare professionals who can address different aspects of the child's condition, including medical, psychological, educational, and social needs.
4. Communicate Effectively:
   - Maintain open and regular communication with the family. Answer their questions, address concerns, and keep them informed about their child's progress.

5. Provide Emotional Support:
    - Offer emotional support to both the child and the family. Connect them with counselors, therapists, or support groups that specialize in dealing with chronic illnesses.
6. Practical Assistance:
    - Help families navigate practical challenges, such as scheduling appointments, managing medications, and coordinating care across different providers.
7. Individualized Care Plans:
    - Develop personalized care plans that take into account the family's preferences, values, and resources. Collaborate to create realistic goals and strategies.
8. Respite Care:
    - Offer respite care options for parents and caregivers to take breaks and recharge. This can provide valuable relief from the constant demands of caregiving.
9. School and Community Support:
    - Collaborate with schools, teachers, and community organizations to ensure that the child's needs are met in educational and social settings.
10. Encourage Self-Care:
    - Encourage parents and caregivers to prioritize their own well-being. Taking care of themselves enables them to better support their child.
11. Financial and Resource Assistance:
    - Help families access financial resources, insurance information, and available support services that can alleviate some of the financial burdens.
12. Normalize Feelings:

- Let families know that it's okay to have mixed feelings, including frustration, sadness, and even moments of joy. Normalizing these feelings can reduce feelings of isolation.

13. Celebrate Achievements:
- Acknowledge and celebrate the child's milestones and achievements, no matter how small. These victories can provide a sense of hope and motivation.

14. Long-Term Support:
- Recognize that support is needed not only at the time of diagnosis but throughout the child's journey with a chronic illness.

Supporting families of children with chronic illnesses requires a compassionate and holistic approach that addresses physical, emotional, and practical needs. By providing a network of care and resources, you can help families navigate the challenges and improve the quality of life for both the child and their loved ones.

Recognizing and Addressing Childhood Anxiety and Depression

Recognizing and addressing childhood anxiety and depression is crucial for promoting the mental health and well-being of children. Anxiety and depression are common mental health conditions that can affect children of all ages. Early intervention and support are key to helping children manage these challenges effectively. Here's how to recognize and address childhood anxiety and depression:

Recognizing Childhood Anxiety:

1. Excessive Worry: Children with anxiety may exhibit excessive worry about various aspects of their lives, such as school performance, relationships, and personal safety.
2. Physical Symptoms: Anxiety can manifest as physical symptoms like headaches, stomachaches, muscle tension, and restlessness.
3. Avoidance Behavior: Children with anxiety may avoid situations or activities that trigger their anxiety.
4. Overthinking and Perfectionism: Anxiety may lead to overthinking situations, seeking constant reassurance, or perfectionistic tendencies.

Recognizing Childhood Depression:

1. Persistent Sadness: Children with depression may consistently display sadness, irritability, or a lack of interest or pleasure in activities they once enjoyed.

2. Changes in Sleep and Appetite: Depression can affect sleep patterns, leading to difficulties falling asleep or sleeping excessively. Changes in appetite and weight may also occur.
3. Low Energy and Fatigue: Children with depression may experience low energy levels and fatigue, which can impact their ability to engage in daily activities.
4. Withdrawal: Depression can lead to social withdrawal, isolation from friends and family, and a lack of interest in social interactions.

Addressing Childhood Anxiety and Depression:

1. Open Communication: Encourage open conversations with your child. Let them know that it's okay to express their feelings and that you're there to listen and support them.
2. Professional Help: If you suspect anxiety or depression, seek help from a mental health professional, such as a child psychologist or psychiatrist, who specializes in working with children.
3. Provide Reassurance: Offer reassurance to your child and let them know that their feelings are valid. Avoid minimizing or dismissing their emotions.
4. Establish Routine: A consistent daily routine can provide a sense of stability and predictability, which can help reduce anxiety and depression.
5. Encourage Healthy Habits: Promote regular exercise, balanced nutrition, and adequate sleep, as these factors contribute to overall mental well-being.
6. Limit Stressors: Reduce unnecessary stressors in your child's life and create a supportive and nurturing environment.
7. Teach Coping Skills: Help your child learn healthy coping strategies, such as deep breathing, mindfulness, and positive self-talk.

8. Involve School: Collaborate with teachers and school staff to create a supportive environment at school. They can be allies in addressing anxiety and depression.
9. Consider Therapy: Cognitive-behavioral therapy (CBT) and other evidence-based therapies can be effective in treating childhood anxiety and depression.
10. Model Healthy Behavior: Be a positive role model by practicing self-care, managing stress, and demonstrating healthy ways of coping with challenges.

Remember that each child is unique, and the approach to addressing anxiety and depression may vary. It's essential to provide unconditional love, support, and patience as your child works through their emotions. If you're concerned about your child's mental health, consult a professional for guidance and assistance.

Child Trauma and Post-Traumatic Stress Disorder (PTSD)

Child trauma refers to an event or series of events that are distressing, overwhelming, and potentially harmful to a child's physical or emotional well-being. Trauma can have a significant impact on a child's psychological and emotional development. Post-Traumatic Stress Disorder (PTSD) is a mental health condition that can develop in some children and adolescents after experiencing or witnessing a traumatic event. Here's an overview of child trauma and PTSD:

Child Trauma:

1. Types of Trauma: Child trauma can result from various experiences, including physical abuse, sexual abuse, neglect, accidents, natural disasters, violence, loss of a loved one, medical procedures, and more.
2. Reactions to Trauma: Children may respond to trauma with a range of reactions, including fear, anxiety, nightmares, flashbacks, withdrawal, behavioral changes, aggression, emotional numbing, and physical symptoms.
3. Long-Term Impact: If not addressed, trauma can lead to emotional and psychological difficulties, such as anxiety disorders, depression, behavioral problems, and difficulties in relationships.

Post-Traumatic Stress Disorder (PTSD) in Children:

1. Symptoms: Children with PTSD may experience

intrusive thoughts, nightmares, flashbacks, avoiding reminders of the traumatic event, changes in mood, irritability, difficulty sleeping, and hyperarousal (being easily startled or on edge).

2. Diagnosis: A diagnosis of PTSD in children involves the presence of specific symptoms over a certain period and their impact on the child's daily functioning.

3. Triggers: Certain cues or reminders related to the traumatic event can trigger intense emotional and physical reactions in children with PTSD.

4. Co-occurring Conditions: Children with PTSD may also experience other mental health conditions, such as depression, anxiety disorders, and substance abuse.

Addressing Child Trauma and PTSD:

1. Safety and Stability: Creating a safe and stable environment is crucial for helping children cope with trauma. Establish routines and provide consistent support.

2. Therapeutic Interventions: Evidence-based therapies such as trauma-focused cognitive-behavioral therapy (TF-CBT) and play therapy can help children process trauma and develop coping skills.

3. Supportive Relationships: Foster nurturing relationships with caregivers, family members, teachers, and friends. Supportive relationships can help buffer the effects of trauma.

4. Avoid Re-traumatization: Be cautious about exposing the child to reminders of the traumatic event. Gradual exposure and desensitization should be guided by a mental health professional.

5. Open Communication: Encourage the child to express their feelings and thoughts about the traumatic event. Offer a nonjudgmental and empathetic listening ear.

6. Professional Help: Consult with a mental health

professional specializing in trauma and child psychology to assess and develop an appropriate treatment plan.

7. Family Involvement: Involve family members in the child's healing process, as family support is crucial for recovery.

8. Educate and Validate: Educate the child about trauma reactions and provide validation for their emotions. Normalize their responses as normal reactions to an abnormal event.

9. Mindfulness and Relaxation Techniques: Teach relaxation techniques, deep breathing exercises, and mindfulness practices to help the child manage anxiety and stress.

10. Monitor Progress: Keep track of the child's progress and any changes in symptoms. Adjust interventions as needed based on their response.

Addressing child trauma and PTSD requires a compassionate and patient approach. Seek guidance from mental health professionals who specialize in trauma and child psychology to ensure appropriate support and intervention for the child's healing journey.

Building Resilience and Coping Skills in Children

Building resilience and coping skills in children is essential for helping them navigate challenges, setbacks, and difficult emotions. Resilience enables children to adapt, bounce back from adversity, and develop a positive outlook on life. Here are strategies to foster resilience and teach coping skills to children:

1. Foster a Supportive Environment:

- Provide a safe and nurturing home environment where children feel loved, valued, and supported by caregivers and family members.
- Encourage open communication and create a space where children can express their feelings and concerns without fear of judgment.

2. Teach Problem-Solving:

- Help children develop problem-solving skills by discussing challenges and brainstorming possible solutions together.
- Encourage them to break down problems into smaller steps and explore different approaches to finding solutions.

3. Model Resilience:

- Model positive coping strategies and resilience in your own life. Children learn by observing how adults handle stress and challenges.

4. Develop Emotional Intelligence:

- Teach children to identify and understand their emotions. Discuss different emotions, their causes, and healthy ways to express them.

5. Encourage Positive Self-Talk:

- Teach children to replace negative self-talk with positive affirmations and thoughts. Help them recognize and challenge irrational or negative beliefs.

6. Build Social Skills:

- Encourage children to build positive relationships with peers and adults. Strong social connections provide emotional support during difficult times.

7. Encourage Healthy Habits:

- Promote physical well-being through regular exercise, balanced nutrition, and adequate sleep. A healthy body supports emotional resilience.

8. Mindfulness and Relaxation:

- Introduce mindfulness techniques, deep breathing exercises, and relaxation activities to help children manage stress and anxiety.

9. Encourage Hobbies and Interests:

- Support children in pursuing hobbies and activities they enjoy. Engaging in enjoyable activities can serve as a positive distraction and source of joy.

10. Problem-Focused Coping: - Teach children to take active steps to address the challenges they face. Help them break down problems and work on finding solutions.

11. Emotion-Focused Coping: - Teach children healthy ways to

cope with their emotions, such as talking to a trusted adult, engaging in creative outlets, or engaging in physical activity.

12. Encourage Flexibility: - Help children develop the ability to adapt to changing circumstances and adjust their goals when necessary.

13. Set Realistic Expectations: - Teach children that setbacks are a normal part of life and that they can learn and grow from challenges.

14. Encourage Positivity: - Foster a positive outlook by encouraging children to focus on their strengths, achievements, and things they are grateful for.

15. Provide Guidance: - Offer guidance and support when children face challenges. Help them break down big tasks into manageable steps.

Building resilience and coping skills takes time and consistent effort. As caregivers, parents, and educators, you play a vital role in helping children develop these important life skills. By teaching resilience and coping strategies, you empower children to face adversity with confidence and navigate life's ups and downs in a healthy and constructive way.

Adolescent Development and Puberty

Adolescent development is a period of significant physical, cognitive, emotional, and social changes that occur during the transition from childhood to adulthood. Puberty is a central aspect of adolescent development, marked by the maturation of reproductive and secondary sexual characteristics. Here's an overview of adolescent development and puberty:

Adolescent Development:

1. Physical Changes: Adolescents experience growth spurts, changes in body composition, and the development of secondary sexual characteristics, such as breast development in girls and facial hair growth in boys.
2. Cognitive Changes: Adolescents develop more advanced cognitive abilities, including abstract thinking, problem-solving, and critical thinking. They become more capable of understanding complex ideas and considering multiple perspectives.
3. Emotional Changes: Adolescents experience intense emotions and may struggle with mood swings. They are developing a sense of identity and self-concept, leading to exploration and self-discovery.
4. Social Changes: Peer relationships become more important during adolescence. Adolescents seek to establish their own identity apart from their family and form closer bonds with friends.
5. Independence: Adolescents strive for greater independence, autonomy, and decision-making. They may challenge authority as they seek to establish their

own values and beliefs.

6. Risk-Taking Behavior: Adolescents are more likely to engage in risky behaviors due to a combination of biological changes and a desire for novelty and sensation-seeking.

Puberty:

1. Onset of Puberty: Puberty typically begins between the ages of 9 and 14 for girls and between 11 and 16 for boys. It is triggered by hormonal changes in the body.

2. Physical Changes in Girls: Girls experience breast development, growth of pubic hair, widening of hips, and the onset of menstruation.

3. Physical Changes in Boys: Boys experience growth of facial and body hair, deepening of the voice, growth of the testes, and an increase in muscle mass.

4. Hormonal Changes: The release of sex hormones (estrogen in girls and testosterone in boys) leads to the development of sexual characteristics and reproductive maturation.

5. Psychological Impact: Puberty can lead to body image concerns, self-esteem issues, and changes in mood due to hormonal fluctuations.

Supporting Adolescents:

1. Open Communication: Create an environment where adolescents feel comfortable discussing their thoughts, concerns, and questions about puberty and other changes.

2. Education: Provide accurate and age-appropriate information about puberty and sexual development. Help them understand the changes their bodies are undergoing.

3. Respect Privacy: Adolescents value their privacy. Respect their boundaries while also being available for

guidance when needed.

4. Healthy Habits: Encourage healthy lifestyle choices, including balanced nutrition, regular exercise, adequate sleep, and stress management.

5. Positive Role Models: Model healthy behaviors and attitudes around body image, self-esteem, relationships, and responsible decision-making.

6. Empathy and Validation: Validate their emotions and experiences, even if you don't fully understand. Adolescents may struggle with self-identity and self-acceptance.

7. Mental Health: Monitor emotional well-being and address any signs of depression, anxiety, or other mental health concerns promptly.

8. Sex Education: Provide comprehensive and accurate sex education that includes information about safe sex, consent, and healthy relationships.

Adolescent development and puberty are dynamic and individual processes. Being supportive, providing accurate information, and maintaining open communication can help adolescents navigate these changes with confidence and resilience.

Adolescent Health Screenings and Preventive Care

Adolescent health screenings and preventive care are essential components of ensuring the well-being and development of adolescents. Regular health checkups, screenings, and discussions with healthcare providers help identify potential health issues early, provide guidance on healthy behaviors, and promote overall adolescent health. Here are some key aspects of adolescent health screenings and preventive care:

1. Comprehensive Health Checkups:

- Adolescents should have regular comprehensive health checkups with a healthcare provider, such as a pediatrician, family physician, or adolescent medicine specialist.
- These checkups typically include a review of medical history, physical examination, and discussions about lifestyle, nutrition, physical activity, mental health, and sexual health.

2. Vaccinations:

- Ensure that adolescents are up-to-date on recommended vaccinations, including those for tetanus, diphtheria, pertussis, human papillomavirus (HPV), meningitis, and influenza.

3. Vision and Hearing Screenings:

- Regular vision and hearing screenings can identify

any issues that may impact school performance, social interactions, and overall well-being.

4. Blood Pressure Screening:

- Regular blood pressure measurements help identify and manage hypertension, a condition that can have long-term health implications.

5. Body Mass Index (BMI) Measurement:

- BMI measurement helps assess whether adolescents are within a healthy weight range. Healthcare providers can offer guidance on nutrition and physical activity based on BMI.

6. Cholesterol Screening:

- Cholesterol screening may be recommended for adolescents with certain risk factors, such as a family history of heart disease or obesity.

7. Diabetes Screening:

- Adolescents with risk factors for diabetes, such as obesity or a family history, may be screened for type 2 diabetes.

8. Mental Health Assessment:

- Screening for mental health conditions, such as depression, anxiety, and eating disorders, is important. Adolescents may also discuss stress, peer relationships, and emotional well-being during checkups.

9. Sexual Health Discussions:

- Adolescents should have open discussions with healthcare providers about sexual health, safe sex practices, contraception, and sexually transmitted infections (STIs).

10. Substance Use Assessment: - Healthcare providers may ask about substance use, such as alcohol, tobacco, and drugs, to identify any potential issues and provide guidance.

11. Injury Prevention Education: - Adolescents should receive education about injury prevention, including seat belt use, helmet safety, and avoiding risky behaviors.

12. Nutrition and Physical Activity Guidance: - Healthcare providers can offer guidance on maintaining a balanced diet and engaging in regular physical activity to promote overall health.

13. Confidentiality and Privacy: - Adolescents may have concerns about confidentiality. Healthcare providers should explain privacy policies and encourage open communication.

14. Collaborative Care: - Adolescent health screenings involve collaboration between healthcare providers, parents, and adolescents themselves to ensure comprehensive care.

Regular health screenings and preventive care provide opportunities to address health concerns early, promote healthy behaviors, and empower adolescents to make informed decisions about their health. Encourage open communication and a supportive environment where adolescents can discuss their health and well-being with confidence.

Addressing Adolescent Substance Abuse and Mental Health

Addressing adolescent substance abuse and mental health issues is crucial for promoting the well-being and healthy development of young individuals. Adolescence is a vulnerable period during which teenagers may face pressures, stressors, and experimentation that can lead to substance use and mental health challenges. Here are strategies for addressing these concerns:

1. Education and Awareness:

- Provide comprehensive education about the risks of substance abuse and the importance of mental health.
- Raise awareness about the potential consequences of substance use, including its impact on physical health, mental well-being, relationships, and future opportunities.

2. Open Communication:

- Create an environment where adolescents feel comfortable discussing their feelings, concerns, and experiences without fear of judgment.
- Encourage open dialogue about substance use, stressors, and mental health challenges.

3. Destigmatize Mental Health:

- Normalize conversations about mental health and reduce stigma by discussing mental health as a part of overall well-being.

- Emphasize that seeking help for mental health concerns is a sign of strength and self-care.

4. Recognize Warning Signs:

- Be aware of warning signs of substance abuse and mental health issues, such as changes in behavior, academic performance, social interactions, and mood.

5. Provide Resources:

- Offer information about resources available for adolescents who are struggling with substance abuse or mental health challenges, such as helplines, support groups, and mental health professionals.

6. Early Intervention:

- Address substance abuse and mental health concerns as early as possible to prevent escalation and promote effective intervention.

7. Professional Help:

- Consult mental health professionals who specialize in working with adolescents if you suspect substance abuse or mental health issues.
- Mental health professionals can conduct assessments, provide therapy, and offer guidance on treatment options.

8. Family Involvement:

- Involve family members in the process of addressing substance abuse and mental health concerns. Family support is crucial for recovery.

9. Peer Support:

- Encourage adolescents to connect with peers who promote healthy behaviors and positive coping strategies.

10. Coping Skills: - Teach adolescents healthy coping strategies to manage stress, anxiety, and emotional challenges. These can include mindfulness, relaxation techniques, and engaging in hobbies.

11. Positive Reinforcement: - Reinforce positive behaviors and achievements to boost self-esteem and motivation to make healthy choices.

12. Limit Access to Substances: - Monitor and limit access to substances that can be abused, such as alcohol, prescription medications, and illicit drugs.

13. Create Healthy Routines: - Encourage a balanced lifestyle with regular physical activity, sufficient sleep, and a healthy diet. These factors contribute to both mental and physical well-being.

Addressing adolescent substance abuse and mental health issues requires a collaborative effort involving parents, caregivers, educators, healthcare professionals, and the adolescents themselves. By providing support, resources, and open communication, we can help adolescents make informed choices and develop healthy coping strategies for life's challenges.

Childproofing the Home and Ensuring Safety

Childproofing the home is essential to create a safe environment for infants and young children. It involves taking precautions to prevent accidents and injuries that can occur due to common household hazards. Here's a comprehensive guide to childproofing the home and ensuring safety:

1. Baby-Proofing Basics:

- Install safety gates at the top and bottom of stairs to prevent falls.
- Use outlet covers to prevent children from inserting objects into electrical outlets.
- Keep small objects, toys, and choking hazards out of reach.

2. Kitchen Safety:

- Use stove knob covers to prevent children from turning on burners.
- Store sharp objects, cleaning supplies, and potentially toxic items in locked cabinets.
- Use stove guards to prevent accidental burns.

3. Bathroom Safety:

- Lock medicine cabinets and keep medications out of reach.
- Use non-slip mats in the bathtub to prevent slips and falls.

- Keep electrical appliances away from water sources.

4. Window and Blind Safety:

- Install window guards to prevent falls from windows.
- Keep cords from blinds and curtains out of reach to prevent strangulation hazards.

5. Furniture and TV Safety:

- Anchor heavy furniture and TVs to the wall to prevent tipping.
- Use corner protectors to soften sharp edges on furniture.

6. Choking Hazards:

- Regularly check for small objects that could be potential choking hazards and remove them from reach.
- Cut food into small, bite-sized pieces to reduce choking risk.

7. Cord Safety:

- Keep cords from blinds, curtains, and electronics out of reach to prevent strangulation hazards.
- Use cord shorteners or wind cords around hooks to keep them tidy.

8. Poison Prevention:

- Store cleaning supplies, medications, and chemicals in locked cabinets.
- Keep the Poison Control hotline number readily accessible (1-800-222-1222 in the United States).

9. Fire and Burns:

- Install smoke detectors on each floor of the home and test them regularly.
- Keep matches, lighters, and candles out of reach.

10. Electrical Safety: - Cover unused electrical outlets with outlet covers or safety plugs. - Keep cords and electrical devices out of reach or secured with cord organizers.

11. Door Safety: - Install door stoppers or pinch guards to prevent fingers from getting caught in doors.

12. Furniture Safety: - Ensure furniture is stable and not wobbly to prevent tipping. - Avoid placing heavy items on top of furniture that could be easily pulled down.

13. Supervision: - Constant supervision is crucial, especially for infants and toddlers. Never leave them unattended, even for a short time.

14. Create a Safe Play Area: - Designate a safe play area where children can explore without access to hazards. - Use playpens, play yards, or baby gates to create a secure space.

15. Regular Checkups: - Regularly assess the childproofing measures in your home as your child grows and becomes more mobile.

Childproofing the home requires a proactive approach to identifying and addressing potential hazards. Regularly assess your home from a child's perspective and make adjustments to ensure their safety. Remember that no childproofing strategy is foolproof, so continuous supervision and education about safety are also crucial components of keeping children safe at home.

Preventing Childhood Accidents and Injuries

Preventing childhood accidents and injuries is a top priority for parents and caregivers. Children are naturally curious and explorative, so it's important to take proactive measures to create a safe environment and teach them about safety. Here are tips to help prevent childhood accidents and injuries:

1. Supervision:

   - Supervise children at all times, especially infants, toddlers, and young children. Even a momentary distraction can lead to accidents.

2. Childproof the Home:

   - Childproof your home by securing furniture, using safety gates, covering outlets, and storing hazardous items out of reach.

3. Use Safety Gear:

   - Ensure children wear appropriate safety gear such as helmets when riding bikes, scooters, or skateboards.

4. Road Safety:

   - Teach children to look both ways before crossing the street and to use designated crosswalks.
   - Hold hands with young children when walking near traffic.

5. Water Safety:

- Never leave children unattended near water, whether it's a bathtub, pool, or any body of water.
- Install pool fences and covers, and teach children to swim at an appropriate age.

6. Kitchen Safety:

- Keep hot items out of reach and use stove knob covers to prevent burns.
- Store sharp objects and cleaning supplies in locked cabinets.

7. Fire Safety:

- Install smoke detectors on each floor of the home and test them regularly.
- Create a fire escape plan and practice it with your family.

8. Choking Hazards:

- Keep small objects, coins, and small toy parts out of reach, especially for infants and toddlers.
- Cut food into small, manageable pieces to reduce choking risk.

9. Poison Prevention:

- Lock away cleaning supplies, medications, and chemicals in cabinets with safety locks.
- Label poisonous items clearly and store them out of reach.

10. Car Safety: - Use appropriate car seats, booster seats, or seat belts for children based on their age, weight, and height. - Never leave children unattended in a parked car, even for a short time.

11. Toy Safety: - Choose age-appropriate toys without small parts that can be swallowed. - Regularly inspect toys for wear and tear,

and discard broken toys.

12. Falls Prevention: - Use safety gates at the top and bottom of stairs to prevent falls. - Install window guards to prevent falls from windows.

13. Sports and Activities: - Ensure children wear protective gear when participating in sports and activities. - Teach them proper techniques and safety rules.

14. Teach Safe Behaviors: - Teach children about stranger danger, fire safety, pedestrian safety, and how to dial emergency numbers.

15. Stay Informed: - Stay informed about current safety guidelines and best practices for preventing childhood accidents.

Preventing childhood accidents and injuries requires a combination of vigilance, education, and creating a safe environment. By being proactive and consistently emphasizing safety, you can significantly reduce the risk of accidents and help children grow up in a secure and nurturing environment.

Advancements in Pediatric Research and Medicine

Advancements in pediatric research and medicine have led to significant improvements in the health and well-being of children. Ongoing research and innovation have contributed to better understanding of pediatric diseases, more effective treatments, and improved preventive measures. Here are some key areas of advancements in pediatric research and medicine:

1. Precision Medicine:

   - Advances in genetic and genomic research have paved the way for personalized treatment approaches. Precision medicine tailors medical care to individual patients' genetic makeup, leading to more targeted and effective treatments.

2. Vaccines and Immunizations:

   - Development of new vaccines and improvements in vaccine delivery have led to better protection against infectious diseases in children. Vaccines have significantly reduced the prevalence of once-common childhood illnesses.

3. Pediatric Surgery and Minimally Invasive Techniques:

   - Advancements in surgical techniques have enabled minimally invasive procedures for a range of pediatric conditions, leading to shorter hospital stays, faster recovery, and reduced scarring.

4. Pediatric Oncology:

- Advances in cancer research have led to improved treatments and survival rates for childhood cancers. Targeted therapies and personalized treatment plans are becoming more common.

5. Pediatric Cardiology:

- Innovations in pediatric cardiology have led to improved diagnosis and treatment of congenital heart defects. Minimally invasive interventions and surgical techniques have improved outcomes.

6. Neonatal Care:

- Advances in neonatal care have contributed to better outcomes for premature and critically ill newborns. Neonatal intensive care units (NICUs) are equipped with advanced medical technologies and therapies.

7. Pediatric Imaging and Diagnostics:

- Advanced imaging technologies, such as MRI and CT scans, provide detailed insights into pediatric conditions, leading to more accurate diagnoses and treatment planning.

8. Stem Cell and Gene Therapies:

- Stem cell and gene therapies offer potential treatments for a variety of pediatric disorders, including genetic conditions and certain types of cancers.

9. Pediatric Neurology:

- Research in pediatric neurology has led to a better understanding of neurological conditions in children, including epilepsy, autism spectrum disorders, and cerebral palsy.

10. Child Mental Health and Development: - Increasing awareness of child mental health has led to improved diagnostic criteria, early interventions, and treatment options for conditions such as ADHD, anxiety, and depression.

11. Telemedicine and Remote Monitoring: - Telemedicine and remote monitoring technologies have expanded access to pediatric care, enabling consultations, follow-ups, and monitoring from a distance.

12. Pediatric Rheumatology and Autoimmune Disorders: - Advances in treatment options for pediatric rheumatology conditions and autoimmune disorders have improved disease management and quality of life.

13. Pediatric Nutrition: - Research on pediatric nutrition has led to improved understanding of dietary needs for children of different ages and conditions, promoting optimal growth and development.

14. Child Safety and Injury Prevention: - Ongoing research on child safety has led to improved safety guidelines, awareness campaigns, and product designs to prevent childhood accidents and injuries.

Advancements in pediatric research and medicine are continually shaping the landscape of healthcare for children. These advancements contribute to better outcomes, improved quality of life, and increased life expectancy for pediatric patients. Ongoing collaboration between researchers, healthcare professionals, and families plays a crucial role in driving these positive changes.

Challenges and Opportunities in Pediatric Healthcare

Pediatric healthcare is a specialized field that comes with both challenges and opportunities. While advancements in medical science have improved child health outcomes, various factors can pose challenges to providing optimal care for children. Here are some key challenges and opportunities in pediatric healthcare:

Challenges:

1. Complexity of Pediatric Conditions: Some pediatric conditions are complex and require specialized care, which can be challenging for healthcare providers to manage effectively.
2. Limited Research and Funding: Pediatric research often receives less funding compared to adult research, leading to a gap in knowledge and treatment options for certain pediatric conditions.
3. Communication and Consent: Communicating medical information to parents and involving children in decision-making can be challenging due to age differences and legal requirements for informed consent.
4. Pediatric Specialists Shortage: There is a shortage of pediatric specialists in some regions, leading to limited access to specialized care for children with complex medical needs.
5. Vulnerable Populations: Children from vulnerable populations, such as low-income families or minority

groups, may face disparities in access to healthcare and quality of care.

6. Transition to Adult Care: Adolescents with chronic conditions need to transition from pediatric to adult care, which can be a complex process involving coordination and adjustment to new healthcare environments.

7. Mental Health Challenges: Identifying and addressing mental health issues in children can be challenging due to stigma, limited mental health resources, and the difficulty of diagnosing certain conditions.

8. Technology Integration: Integrating new technologies into pediatric care, such as telemedicine and electronic health records, requires considerations for privacy, security, and accessibility.

Opportunities:

1. Preventive Care and Education: Educating parents and caregivers about preventive care, nutrition, safety, and healthy habits offers opportunities to promote child health and well-being.

2. Early Intervention: Early intervention for developmental, behavioral, and medical issues can lead to improved outcomes and quality of life for children.

3. Advancements in Research: Advances in genetic research, stem cell therapies, and precision medicine offer opportunities for more targeted and effective treatments for pediatric conditions.

4. Telemedicine: Telemedicine can improve access to care, especially for families in rural or underserved areas, and enable remote consultations with pediatric specialists.

5. Integrated Care: Collaborative care models involving pediatricians, specialists, therapists, and educators can provide comprehensive support for children with complex needs.

6. Mental Health Focus: Increasing awareness about child mental health and providing accessible mental health services can lead to better emotional well-being for children.
7. Family-Centered Care: Engaging families in the care process and considering their preferences and needs can improve patient outcomes and satisfaction.
8. Advocacy and Policy Change: Advocacy efforts can drive policy changes that prioritize pediatric healthcare, research funding, and access to care.
9. Training and Education: Providing ongoing training and education for healthcare professionals in pediatric care can improve the quality of care delivered.
10. Community Engagement: Partnering with schools, community organizations, and local governments can promote child health, safety, and wellness on a broader scale.

Pediatric healthcare presents both challenges that need to be addressed and opportunities to improve the health and well-being of children. By recognizing these challenges and capitalizing on opportunities, healthcare providers, researchers, policymakers, and communities can work together to ensure that children receive the best possible care and support.

Ensuring a Healthy Future for Children Worldwide

Ensuring a healthy future for children worldwide is a shared goal that requires collective efforts from governments, organizations, healthcare professionals, communities, and individuals. Promoting child health and well-being on a global scale involves addressing various challenges and implementing comprehensive strategies. Here are some key areas to focus on for ensuring a healthy future for children worldwide:

1. Universal Healthcare Access:

- Ensure that all children have access to essential healthcare services, including preventive care, immunizations, treatment for illnesses, and maternal and child health services.

2. Malnutrition Prevention and Nutrition Education:

- Address malnutrition by providing adequate nutrition and access to clean water and sanitation facilities.
- Educate parents and caregivers about proper nutrition for children's growth and development.

3. Vaccination Programs:

- Implement and sustain vaccination programs to protect children from preventable diseases and achieve high immunization coverage rates.

4. Maternal and Child Health:

- Ensure access to quality prenatal and maternal care to reduce maternal and infant mortality rates.
- Provide postnatal care and support for new mothers and infants.

5. Education and Awareness:

- Raise awareness about child health issues, including the importance of vaccination, nutrition, hygiene, and safe practices.
- Educate families about recognizing signs of illness and seeking timely medical care.

6. Safe Water and Sanitation:

- Improve access to clean and safe drinking water and sanitation facilities to prevent waterborne diseases and improve overall health.

7. Prevention of Infectious Diseases:

- Implement strategies to prevent the spread of infectious diseases through hygiene practices, proper waste management, and vector control.

8. Maternal and Child Nutrition:

- Promote breastfeeding and provide access to nutritious foods to support children's physical and cognitive development.

9. Early Childhood Development:

- Invest in early childhood development programs that provide children with quality education, play, and stimulation for healthy brain development.

10. Child Protection and Safety: - Develop and enforce child protection policies to prevent child labor, exploitation, abuse, and trafficking. - Promote safe environments and injury prevention

measures for children.

11. Mental Health Support: - Integrate mental health services into primary healthcare to address emotional and psychological well-being from an early age.

12. Adolescent Health Services: - Provide comprehensive health services and education for adolescents, including sexual and reproductive health, mental health support, and substance abuse prevention.

13. Research and Innovation: - Invest in research to understand and address the unique health needs of children worldwide, including infectious diseases, malnutrition, and developmental disorders.

14. Global Partnerships: - Collaborate with international organizations, governments, NGOs, and community groups to share resources, expertise, and best practices.

15. Advocacy and Policy Change: - Advocate for policies that prioritize child health, education, and well-being on national and global levels.

Ensuring a healthy future for children worldwide requires a comprehensive and multidimensional approach. It involves addressing immediate health concerns, promoting education and awareness, and working together to create supportive environments for children to thrive. By prioritizing child health and well-being, we can contribute to a brighter future for all children, regardless of their geographic location or socioeconomic background.

Embracing the Journey of Pediatrics

Embracing the journey of pediatrics is a rewarding and impactful path that involves caring for the health and well-being of children from infancy through adolescence. As pediatric healthcare providers, educators, parents, and caregivers, this journey comes with its challenges, joys, and opportunities to make a positive difference in the lives of young individuals. Here are some aspects to consider when embracing the journey of pediatrics:

1. Compassion and Empathy:

- Children are unique individuals with their own needs and emotions. Embrace empathy and compassion as you provide care and support tailored to each child's personality and circumstances.

2. Lifelong Impact:

- The care you provide during childhood can have a lasting impact on a child's overall health and development. Your guidance and support can shape their future well-being.

3. Advocacy for Children:

- Embrace the role of advocate for children's health and well-being. Be their voice in promoting policies, resources, and initiatives that prioritize their needs.

4. Continuous Learning:

- Pediatrics is a field that constantly evolves with new research, treatments, and best practices. Embrace lifelong learning to stay up-to-date and provide the best care possible.

5. Building Relationships:

- Building strong relationships with children and their families is essential. These connections help create a supportive environment for children's growth and development.

6. Celebrating Milestones:

- Celebrate the milestones and achievements of the children you care for, whether it's their first steps, academic accomplishments, or personal growth.

7. Navigating Challenges:

- Pediatric care can present challenges, including medical complexities and emotional needs. Embrace these challenges as opportunities to learn, adapt, and make a positive impact.

8. Embracing Diversity:

- Children come from diverse backgrounds, cultures, and experiences. Embrace cultural competency and inclusivity to provide care that respects and values their uniqueness.

9. Joy of Play and Exploration:

- Embrace the joy of working with children who are naturally curious, playful, and full of wonder. Engage in activities that promote their physical, cognitive, and emotional development.

10. Witnessing Resilience: - Children often show remarkable resilience in the face of illness, adversity, and challenges. Embrace the privilege of witnessing their strength and growth.

11. Contributing to Future Generations: - By providing quality pediatric care, you contribute to the well-being of future generations, making a positive impact on families and communities.

12. Fostering Health Habits: - Embrace the opportunity to teach children and families about healthy habits that can have lifelong benefits, from nutrition and exercise to emotional well-being.

13. Preventive Focus: - Embrace the preventive aspect of pediatric care by promoting immunizations, safety measures, and early intervention to prevent health issues.

14. Creating Safe Spaces: - Create environments where children feel safe, valued, and heard, fostering their trust and comfort in seeking medical care.

15. Celebrating Milestones: - Celebrate your own journey in pediatrics and the impact you've had on the lives of the children and families you've cared for.

Embracing the journey of pediatrics is a privilege that allows you to play a vital role in nurturing the health, development, and happiness of children. Your dedication and commitment contribute to building a healthier and brighter future for generations to come.

Empowering Parents and Caregivers in Child Health

Empowering parents and caregivers in child health is essential for promoting the well-being and development of children. When parents and caregivers are informed, confident, and engaged in their child's health, they can make informed decisions, provide effective care, and create a supportive environment for the child's growth. Here are ways to empower parents and caregivers in child health:

1. Education and Information:

- Provide accurate and clear information about child health, development, and common childhood conditions.
- Offer resources, brochures, and online materials to help parents understand their child's needs.

2. Open Communication:

- Foster open and transparent communication between healthcare providers and parents. Listen to their concerns and address their questions.

3. Shared Decision-Making:

- Involve parents in the decision-making process regarding their child's healthcare, treatment options, and interventions.

4. Teach Basic First Aid and Safety:

- Educate parents about basic first aid skills and safety measures to prevent accidents and respond to emergencies.

5. Encourage Questions:

- Encourage parents to ask questions during healthcare visits and seek clarification on any doubts they may have.

6. Parent Support Groups:

- Connect parents with support groups where they can share experiences, exchange information, and receive emotional support.

7. Developmental Milestones:

- Educate parents about developmental milestones, helping them recognize when their child is on track or may need additional support.

8. Nutrition and Healthy Habits:

- Provide guidance on nutrition, healthy eating habits, and physical activity for the child's optimal growth and well-being.

9. Stress Management and Self-Care:

- Offer parents strategies for managing stress, practicing self-care, and maintaining their own well-being.

10. Mental Health Awareness: - Raise awareness about child mental health and provide guidance on recognizing signs of emotional well-being issues.

11. Active Involvement: - Encourage parents to actively participate in their child's healthcare visits, treatment plans, and therapy sessions.

12. Continuity of Care: - Facilitate consistent healthcare by providing information about follow-up appointments, medications, and treatment plans.

13. Encourage Advocacy: - Empower parents to advocate for their child's health and well-being within healthcare settings and in their community.

14. Online Resources: - Offer online platforms, websites, or apps with reliable information about child health, development, and parenting tips.

15. Tailored Guidance: - Provide guidance that considers the unique needs and circumstances of each child and family.

Empowering parents and caregivers in child health creates a partnership that benefits both the child and the family. When parents are confident in their ability to care for their child's health and well-being, children are more likely to thrive, develop positive health habits, and achieve their full potential. By fostering collaboration, communication, and education, healthcare providers can play a crucial role in empowering parents and caregivers to become effective advocates for their children's health.

Encouragement for Further Exploration and Advocacy for Child Health

Exploring and advocating for child health is a meaningful and impactful journey that can make a positive difference in the lives of children and their families. Your efforts to learn, raise awareness, and advocate for child health can contribute to healthier communities and a brighter future for the next generation. Here's some encouragement to further explore and advocate for child health:

1. A Path of Impact:

- By delving into child health, you're choosing a path that has a profound impact on children's lives. Your actions can shape their well-being, development, and opportunities.

2. Lifelong Learning:

- Child health is a field that continuously evolves. Each new piece of knowledge you gain contributes to your ability to provide effective care and advocate for change.

3. Be the Voice:

- Children need advocates who can raise awareness about their unique health needs, ensuring that their voices are heard and their rights are protected.

4. Empowerment Through Knowledge:

- Knowledge is empowering. The more you learn about

child health, the better equipped you are to make informed decisions and guide others.

5. Catalyst for Change:

- Your advocacy efforts can act as a catalyst for policy changes, better resources, and improved healthcare access for children and families.

6. Collaboration and Networking:

- Exploring child health allows you to connect with like-minded individuals, organizations, and professionals who share your passion for making a difference.

7. Influencing Future Generations:

- Your advocacy work can have a ripple effect, influencing the health and well-being of not only the current generation but also future generations to come.

8. Making a Difference Locally and Globally:

- Whether you're advocating in your local community or on a global scale, your efforts contribute to a larger movement toward child health and well-being.

9. Addressing Disparities: - Advocating for child health can address health disparities and inequalities, ensuring that all children have access to quality care.

10. Amplify Parental Voices: - Your advocacy can amplify the voices of parents and caregivers who may need support, resources, and information to care for their children effectively.

11. Inspiring Change: - Your commitment to child health can inspire others to get involved, creating a collective effort to improve the lives of children.

12. Future Innovations: - As you explore child health, you may contribute to innovations, research, and initiatives that shape the

future of pediatric healthcare.

13. Advocacy as a Lifelong Commitment: - Advocating for child health is a lifelong commitment that aligns with your values and contributes to the betterment of society.

14. Empowering Families: - Your advocacy efforts can empower families to take an active role in their children's health and well-being, fostering a culture of proactive care.

15. Be a Changemaker: - Through your exploration and advocacy, you become a changemaker who sparks positive shifts in policies, attitudes, and outcomes related to child health.

Remember that every effort, no matter how small, contributes to the greater cause of child health. Your passion and dedication can inspire positive change and contribute to a healthier, happier, and more equitable future for children worldwide. Your advocacy matters, and your journey is one of significance and purpose.

www.ingramcontent.com/pod-product-compliance
Lightning Source LLC
Chambersburg PA
CBHW072216290526
45794CB00004B/1771